FIVE FINGERS:

The Story of the Free Medical Clinic
of America,
Knoxville, Tennessee

By

Tom Kim, MD

As told to

Ed Cate

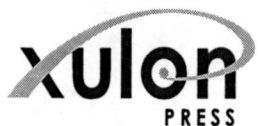

Copyright © 2009
by Tom Kim, MD as told to Ed Cate

Five Fingers
by Tom Kim, MD as told to Ed Cate

Printed in the United States of America

ISBN 9781615793990

All rights reserved solely by the author. The author guarantees all contents are original and do not infringe upon the legal rights of any other person or work. No part of this book may be reproduced in any form without the permission of the author. The views expressed in this book are not necessarily those of the publisher.

www.xulonpress.com

Dear Cal.

One good deed A day
4-16-10

[signature]

For Dr. Bong Oh Kim and Mrs. Soon Bin Kim
With my love and respect

ACKNOWLEDGEMENTS

I would like to acknowledge and thank the true heroes of this story— the many individuals who made the Free Clinic possible. Without their help, the Free Clinic, as we know it today, would still be just a dream. They have my sincere admiration and gratitude.

As early as 1993, Congressman Jimmy Duncan recognized my work with the uninsured and has been an enthusiastic sponsor ever since. Randy Tyree, former Mayor of Knoxville, has supported the clinic for many years. The current Mayors of Knox County and Knoxville, Mike Ragsdale and Bill Haslam respectively, have assisted the 2005 expansion of the Free Clinic in many ways. Special thanks go to Knox County Commissioners Paul Pinkston, Mike Brown, and former Commissioner John Mills who saw the clinic as an integral part of constituent service. I am grateful for the help and advice provided by many other local and state elected and appointed officials.

Five Fingers

Dale Collins, President and CEO of Baptist Health System, was my initial community contact early in 2005. He has stayed the course and continues to support our efforts. He also began the clinic's relationship with the Baptist Health System Foundation, and without their shepherding there would be no Free Clinic today. Executive Director & CEO, Terry Morgan, led the way. Without Donna Edwards, Eunice Goodwin, Dena Mashburn, Jo Ann Parker, Pat Scott, Wright Tisdale, and Erin Upshaw handling details, I doubt the "Nike Clinic" would have ever opened.

Baptist Health System also provided free diagnostic testing. Since Baptist's 2008 merger into Mercy Health Partners, this generous support has continued. Appreciation goes to Jerry Askew, Ph.D., Mercy's Senior Vice President for External Affairs, who ensured the transition went smoothly. Laboratory Corporation of America has provided free lab testing since the clinic opened and their unstinting generosity is acknowledged.

The Free Clinic was extremely fortunate to have wonderful local media support. Bill Williams, the "Dean" of Knoxville TV News Anchors, Bruce Hartmann, Publisher of the Knoxville News Sentinel, and Kristi Nelson, the Sentinel's medical beat reporter deserve particular mention. Credit also goes to the management and staff of WATE-TV, WBIR-TV, and WVLT-TV, along with radio stations WJBZ-FM and WRJZ-JOY 62.

Five Fingers

The founding board members of the Free Clinic were: Judy Bacon, Penny Bandy, Dale Collins, Dale Keasling, Wayne Kline, Bo Shafer, and Bill Williams. They have served the clinic well and have my thanks. In addition to serving as Chair, Wayne Kline has given generously of his time and legal expertise. His hard work and wise counsel have ensured the Free Clinic is on a firm organizational foundation.

Over the years, almost 175 volunteers have served the Free Clinic in some capacity. Because they deserve special recognition for launching the clinic, the doctors, nurses, and office workers who served in the first 90 days are recognized below:

Doctors: Michael Bernard, William Bolin, Richard Brinner, Monte Broome, Jeffrey Brown, Leonard Brown, Ron Bryan, Brantly Burns, Ivan Cooper, James Cox, Evelyne Davidson, Elise Denneny, James Denneny, Albert Ebenezer, Erik Geibig, John Goodwin, Randal Graham, Mike Helton, Casey Hewgley, John Howard, James Hudgens, Hugh Hyatt, Sunil John, Edward Kim, Michael Kropilak, Jenifer Kurtz, Henry Lau, Richard Lee, David Martin, Bill Merwin, Gregory Midis, Tom Miller, Frank Murchison, Jr., Pat O'Brien, Jason Ozment, Casey Paige, Jon Parham, David Rankin, Jim Reynolds, Toivo Rist, Scott Rosenbloom, John Royer, Stephen Russell, Deaton Smith, Jerry Sanders, Wayne Stuart, David Stockton, Bill Sullivan, Bob Sullivan, Hiroshi Toyohara, Mark Turner, Greg Wheatley, Ceeccy

Yang, Ron Yatteau, Jay Young, Richard Young, and Kevin Zirkle.

Nurses: Libby Amero, Elain Anderson, Susan Beara, Barbara Burber, Joy Carleston, Bonnie DiMolfetta, Mary Farmer, Felicia Gaddi, Jan Garmbu, Gail Harbin, Tracy Hicks, Pam Hutchens, Christy Kidwell, Ramore Kimmins, Kathy McGraw, Kim Menard, Martha Mynatt, Penny Reagan, Kristy Reed, Sandy Rysewyk, Vickie Scalf, Norma Seals, Joan Sitton, Kathy Smith, Cheryl Sowdu, and Lynn Whitaker.

Office Volunteers: Nell Afaro, Rita Brooks, Norma Jean Burnett, Ed Cate, Nancy Cate, June Cely, Carol Clifton, Marinel Edwards, Girall Evans, Mary June Faulk, June Gibbs, Jim Gill, Rebecca Grubert, Pam Harwell, Rebecca Husein, Shelia Jacobstein, Brenda Jordan, Joan & John Leonarz, Shirley McCroskey, Lorraine McPherson, Laura Lee Needham, Jean Perry, Joyce Rasar, Beth Sams, Kimberly Sapp, Susan Schultz, Janis Sims, Dana Sims, Doris Tipton, Margaret Trainer, Kitty VanDuser, Hilda Wampler, Lynne Webb, Robin Williams, Eileen Wilson, Nora Wiser, Mary Lou Witt, Michele Woods, and Mary Jane Spaeth.

I also want to thank the Knoxville community for its support. Randy Overby, retired Alcoa Inc, Dr. John Hawkins, DDS, Alan Frye and Rich Nichols of Vol Market #3, and Yang Ku Woo, CEO/President of S L America Corporation are typical of the grassroots assistance the clinic has enjoyed.

They represent hundreds who have lent a hand in many different ways.

Finally, I want to especially thank my wife Hwa, daughter Kimberly, son Tim, and good friend B Ray Thompson, Jr. They have supported me in this long journey in many special ways and I will never be able to adequately express my love and appreciation.

Tom Kim, MD

TABLE OF CONTENTS

PROLOUGE xv
A KOREAN HILLBILLY 23
THE SERMON 33
LEAP OF FAITH 42
THE MEETING 55
A CHANGE OF PACE 64
TAKING SOME RISKS 73
HELP ALONG THE WAY 84
THE DAYS 103
OPENING DAY 114
THE WEEKS 123
THE YEARS 143
THE LESSONS 164
NOW WHAT? 180
Appendix I – Additional Information 183

PROLOGUE

As the Obama administration prepares to deal with the thorny issue of health care, we can expect the media to spend some time reporting on the current state of affairs. There should be numerous pieces discussing the problem of the millions of Americans who lack ready access to health care. Look for wide ranging estimates of individuals without health insurance that have a median of around fifty million.

There may be arguments about the cause, the exact number, and the best solution to this fiasco, but one point of general agreement seems to be that the need is great. Whether citing the impact of indigent Emergency Room visits, the cost of restorative versus preventative treatment, the human suffering, or any of the other complex associated factors, very few deny there is a crisis and its scope is extensive. For years this need and the desire to do something about it has moved many individuals.

Such was the case in 2005. One doctor in Knoxville, Tennessee decided to do something and to do it quickly. Dr. Tom Kim had practiced medicine in South Knox County, an area with significant economic needs, for over twenty-four years. For twelve of those years he provided free care to working uninsured patients in an after-hours clinic at his office. Though an informal, one-man operation, called The Free Medical Clinic of America, it had provided healthcare to many uninsured folk.

In early 2005, Dr. Kim made a commitment to expand his part-time work to a full time volunteer clinic with multiple doctors. He intended to provide health care for those without health insurance who did not qualify for public assistance. As he sought support for the clinic over the years, he made an appeal that he coined as the "Five Fingers." Like giving a "high five," he encourages like-minded folk to raise five fingers as a reminder of how everyone can begin today to combat the suffering of the uninsured. The five fingers represent one day, one doctor, one patient, one church, and one dollar. For Tom Kim, this is the way to address uninsured health care concerns today.

The one day component means addressing the problem immediately, but also solving it one day at a time. When considering the scope of the problem, it is easy to bury one's head in the sand and say there is no way to solve such a massive task. On the contrary, Kim believes that a single act on a single day, combined with other acts of assistance, will bring about a solution. Do what can be done today and trust it will bear more fruit in the days ahead. To Kim, one day at a time is an organizational principle that works well in many settings.

One doctor means that a large, institutional, or highly organized program is not the only possible solution. If every doctor helps, the solution may be that simple. Dr. Kim does not discount large programs and admires their economy of scale and the higher levels of care they can offer. In fact, his clinic is now one of those larger more structured projects. His point is that every doctor can contribute as an individual or as a member of an organization. Dr. Jack McConnell, the well-known founder of the Volunteers in Medicine Clinic in Hilton Head, South Carolina, agrees in principle when he states, "It [serving the uninsured] can also be achieved by every physician in his office."

And, it is clear when talking to Dr. Kim, that his thinking has expanded the term "doctor" to mean more than just MDs. It has become a figure of speech implying that everyone can and should do something to help. Certainly, doctors are the primary means of delivering health care, but they need many others supporting them to be efficient and effective. So while physicians are at the tip of the spear, the nurses, administrators, and others who support them are necessary parts of the system. "One doctor" includes the many helping hands necessary to make a volunteer health care organization work.

One patient is again an expression of the fact that the fifty or more million Americans without health insurance can only be helped one at a time. Don't focus on the millions that need help. Focus on the one you can help today. "A journey of a thousand miles begins with a single step," and caring for the uninsured begins with a single patient. Find that patient. Find a way to bring the immediate care needed. Encourage them to take their medicine, return for a check-up, quit smoking, lose weight, exercise, and do all the things that build a healthier lifestyle. Support them emotionally and financially if necessary. As the single patients receive help, they will add up to the thousands and eventually the millions.

One church has special meaning to Dr. Kim. Kim added this "finger" because much of the initial support for the clinic came from churches. Presbyterian, Methodist, and Baptist congregations were among the first to respond to his requests for support. (This was due to membership and geographical ties; with Cedar Springs Presbyterian being Dr. Kim's home church, and the others located near the clinic in South Knoxville.) As the clinic grew, many different religious and civic groups asked Kim to speak. His reception at churches of various religions and denominations was universally warm. It was reasonable that he began to see "churches" as a natural source of support.

In his many visits to churches, he developed the habit of scouting out spaces that might serve as part-time clinics. He challenged more than one congregation to start a clinic, if only one day a month. His vision at one time was that every church in Knoxville would have a free clinic, either on its own or in combination with other churches. While this vision has not yet matured in Knoxville, Dr. Kim remains convinced that churches are the most likely sources of support for volunteer clinics. The number of Free Clinic volunteers and supporters from church groups led him to add the fourth finger of one church. It symbolizes that they usually make enthusiastic supporters.

The final finger of "one dollar" acknowledges that many small contributions add up and can sustain a community clinic. A clinic that relies more on volunteer time, small donations, and in-kind support may be stronger in the long run than one receiving a large, one time grant. Seeking only "one dollar" may actually increase sustainability because the clinic is not dependent on a few large donors. Wise foundations understand this and some will not grant start up funds unless the grantee's business plan supports a "going concern." Dr. Kim believes grassroots financial support from the community is essential to a volunteer clinic's success.

When meeting Dr. Kim, expect him to say, "Give me five." He is not looking for a high five, but hopes to hear one day, one doctor, one patient, one church, one dollar. This is his short hand for how to attack the problems of the uninsured in America. It embodies a call to immediate action and not to be afraid to start small. A program that never starts can never grow. One doctor treating one patient each day with the support of one church contributing a small amount can be a giant step in the right direction.

"Five Fingers" is a reminder that committed individuals can do a great deal to solve the plight of the uninsured if they will just act. It does not always take a large well organized, fully funded entity to address the problem. Nor, does everything have to be perfect—in the sense that the best can be the enemy of the good. Thus, this is the story of how one free clinic opened on faith before everything was neatly in place and prospered through commitment, hard work, and constant learning.

Dr. Kim had not solved or anticipated every problem that would be encountered. Mistakes were made, some things could have been done better, and some hard lessons were learned. Yet, a functioning clinic was up and running and serving more than eighty patients a week within six months of the initial idea. At the start, the clinic did not have a board or a business plan. It did not have any grants or other reliable funding. It simply could not wait for those things to be in place. What it did have was a vision, a willingness to learn and grow, good advice, the will to succeed, and eventually a story to tell.

When telling the story of the clinic, it must be made clear that while the clinic operated at some risk, it never took unnecessary chances or sacrificed the highest standards of medical care. The clinic always erred on the side of caution in its medical practice. An arrangement existed with a nearby emergency room to refer immediately any potential emergency cases. In the first months, an MD drew all blood samples—an inefficient use of professional assets, but necessary until adequate procedures and quality control were in place. The clinic medical director reviewed volunteer physician's notes and treatment plans. Since no pediatricians were on site, the clinic would not treat children under sixteen, an unfortunate limitation that continues due to the lack of specialty support.

A final note on terminology: Free Clinic (in capitals), refers to the Free Medical Clinic of America in Knoxville, Tennessee (AKA The Free Medical Clinic - A Christian Ministry). This clinic existed as an informal organization for many years prior to receiving its charter from the State of Tennessee in March 2005. This story tells of its start-up for expanded operations, beginning August 1, 2005, and operations since then.

The Baptist Health System (BHS) is the entity Knoxvillians have known for many years as Baptist Hospital, or Baptist Hospital of East Tennessee. Baptist Health System no longer exists, having merged with another local hospital system and renamed Mercy Health Partners. Due to reorganization, the "Baptist Hospital" that played such a vital role in the Free Clinic story has changed to an outpatient facility called the "Riverside Campus." The Baptist Health System Foundation was the philanthropic arm of Baptist Health System and is referred to as "The Foundation." For the clinic planners and staff, this was a term of endearment as much as a short title.

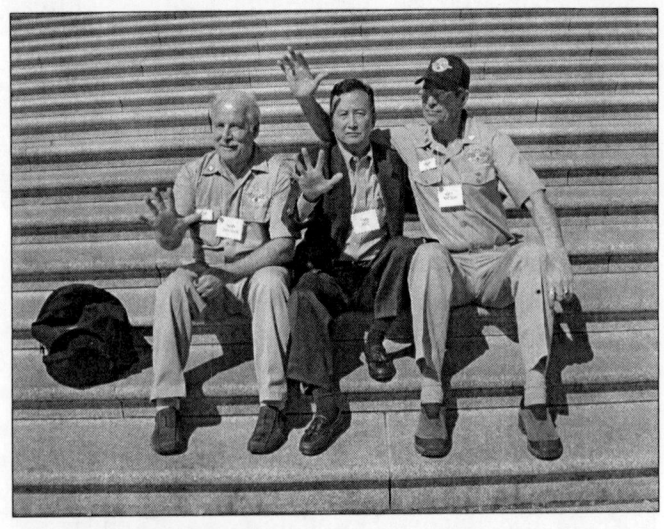

Dr. Kim and Remote Area Medical (RAM) personnel showing "Five Fingers" on the Capitol steps, April 2008. From left to right: Ron Brewer, Tom, and Roy Wilson

A KOREAN HILLBILLY

The story of how one volunteer clinic opened on faith before everything was neatly in place and succeeded is much like the story of the Little Engine That Could. Moving from "I think I can" to "I know I can" is often a tale of how one person's tenacity and commitment are the key to accomplishing what others say is impossible. That is certainly the case with Knoxville's Free Medical Clinic of America. The Free Medical Clinic of America, usually referred to in Knoxville simply as the "Free Clinic," exists largely because of one man – Dr. Tom Kim. He saw a need and decided he must do something big and do it quickly. He envisioned a clinic staffed with volunteers that gave totally free medical care to those in genuine need.

Before covering the details of how he achieved this, it seems important to give some background on Dr. Kim. A number of years and exciting events, that sound more like an action movie script than a Southern internist's biography, formed this exceptional individual's character. The Free Clinic actually has it roots in the turbulent years of the Korean War and the life experiences of a young Korean boy who found a new life in America. In some ways, this narrative explains how a nice Korean boy from a well-educated, privileged family ended up in the hills of East Tennessee providing free medical care to the working uninsured.

Tom Kim was born, December 26, 1944, in Chung Hwa, Korea, now a part of North Korea. His immediate ancestors included a great-grandfather who was a high Provincial official, a grandfather who was a widely respected and beloved Presbyterian minister, and a father who was a practicing physician. The Kims were devout Christians and had ample opportunities to prove their faith during the Japanese occupation of World War Two. Tom's grandfather became renowned among Korean Christians for his resistance to the Japanese and his refusal to compromise his Christian faith.

The end of the Second World War and the Japanese occupation of Korean did not end the trials faced by the Kim family, rather increased them. Korea was divided with a Soviet Union backed communist government under Kim Il Sung in the North and a US supported government under Syngman Rhee in the South. Living in the Communist North placed great pressure on Tom's father because he was a well-known Christian physician. He was twice imprisoned, finally escaping from jail and making his way to the South. The story of his escape is quite exciting. It involved cell mates who were hardened criminals but still aided him and a pursuit through the Mo Rang Bong Mountains. It ended with a clandestine crossing into South Korea. An elder of his grandfather's church arranged the escape. Tom's father hid in a load of charcoal and his mother posed as a helper. After their crossing, Tom's parents stayed temporarily in Seoul.

The 1948 flight of his parents to South Korea left the remaining Kim family in North Korea with Tom's grandmother. The ebb and flow of the Korean War provided the opportunity to reunite the family. As United Nations troops advanced into North Korea, Tom, his siblings, an aunt, and his grandmother, were able to board a train moving troops to the South in the bitter cold of January 1951. They carried only what they wore and had to ride on the open top of the train. Tom recalls his younger brother and himself being tied with a rope so they wouldn't fall. As a six year old, Tom remembers the biting cold, the hunger, and the fear of what might lie ahead, but says he learned that in war, "You just leave everything and run."

The reunited family settled for a time in Pusan where both his mother and father worked as civilian medical professionals in a POW camp. In 1952, Tom's father was able to travel to America. This began a long separation of Tom and his father. In 1959 Tom's mother was able to join her husband in the United States. But, it was not until 1961 that the Kim family was reunited. In that year, Tom, along with three brothers, came to America. He had been separated from his mother for two years and from his father for ten.

Five Fingers

Arrival in America did not eliminate all of Tom's problems; it simply changed his immediate concerns. He went from being a top student in middle school dealing with family separation and uncertainty, to being the new kid on the block. The warmth of his newly regained family life did little to lessen the daily struggle with a new language and culture. Moving as his father found better jobs as a physician made the task of becoming part of his new world much more difficult.

Tom spent his first year in the US in New Jersey, with many weekends visiting the small Korean community in New York City and its Korean Church. The language barrier was obvious and enormous to a teenager in a new land. He struggled with improving his English, even trying to live with an American family, an effort that lasted only a month. He did manage to begin his assimilation into a new culture through wrestling, other sports, and extracurricular activities.

His Korean given name was Yoo (pronounced "you"). Mr. Crawford, a caring gym teacher, observed that whenever he called for Yoo all the boys in class turned in response. He suggested Kim use a more distinctive first name. As long as he was picking a new name, it might as well be one associated with a famous American like "Thomas Jefferson" or "Thomas Edison". So, Yoo adopted the anglicized name of "Tom" and has been known as Tom Kim ever since.

Three years in the Gary, Indiana area followed that first year in New Jersey. Again, due to his father's professional moves, Tom attended three different high schools. He spent his senior year at Horace Mann High School in Gary. By now Tom was more a typical American teenager than a Korean newcomer. He was a popular student and accomplished athlete. He never felt any discernible prejudice and remembers being well treated and accepted by his classmates. With a brother and himself as virtually the only Asians in the school, Tom describes his treatment more like a VIP than an outsider. This only increased his love and gratitude for his newfound home of America.

As Tom was immersing himself in his challenging but relatively comfortable new lifestyle, he also began to seriously consider what he would do with his life. His grandfather's ministry and example had profoundly influenced him and he felt some call to mission work. His father's career had also exposed him first hand to the medical profession. So as a young man, Tom Kim saw combining the two as a medical missionary a perfect fit.

Through a church visitor, Tom became interested in Milligan College, a small Christian liberal arts school in Johnson City, Tennessee. Although accepted at the University of Indiana, his medical missionary calling caused him to enroll at Milligan without ever visiting the campus. He thrived at Milligan College. In addition to completing the courses and earning the grades to compete for a medical school slot, Tom was a varsity athlete and involved in numerous extracurricular activities. He wrestled and played tennis. In tennis, he played in the number one spot and was captain of the team. He served as president of four college organizations – Fellowship of Christian Athletes, International Club, Pre-Med Club, and Judo Club. With his Black Belt, Tom was not only president, but a primary instructor in the Judo Club.

Juggling a schedule like this was very stressful. In addition to study, tennis practice, and his service activities, Tom had to diet to make weight for wrestling matches. This often involved losing eight to ten pounds in a week that was a great physical strain for a 130 pound young man. During his senior year, he considered giving up wrestling since constantly dropping weight made it hard to study and he needed good grades to have a shot at medical school. In his own words, he realized "he was not a quitter," and finished four years of college wrestling. Over the years, in times of stress and challenge, he has often looked back to that time and refused to quit when faced with a challenge.

With the advice and assistance of his pre-med advisor, Tom applied to the Indiana University Medical School and was offered a seat in a six year program leading to a dual MD and PhD degree. Since he hoped to return to Korea as a medical missionary as soon as possible, he looked for other options. His father suggested returning to Korea for medical school. In an odd turn of events, Tom felt language would be a barrier to his attending medical school in Korea. Tom Kim was thoroughly "Americanized" by this time. However, knowing The University of Yonsei School of Medicine (Severance Medical School) in Seoul used mainly English textbooks, he applied. He was accepted there as well and now had to make a final decision on a medical school.

He chose Yonsei over Indiana. His choice to return to Korea disappointed his mother. She loved America, had no desire to return to Korea, nor did she want her son to return. Tom remembers his mother crying and begging him not to go. As difficult as the decision was, he laid aside the pleas of his mother because he felt the Lord was leading him back to Korea. It was hard for a youngster in his twenties to leave home and family to boldly follow a dream. Yet just as he had refused to quit wrestling, he decided to take the harder right rather than the easier wrong. The character seen in Tom Kim's adult professional and public service life was molded early.

How life often comes full circle! A decade earlier, Tom had found himself in a strange land struggling with a language he did not fully understand. Now he was back in his native land facing exactly the same circumstances. Medical school was hard and he had no comprehension of most Korean technical terms. Some courses also used many Chinese characters that caused him trouble. He was not afraid of hard work, but asked one professor whose class required long written descriptions for permission to write in English. The professor agreed until his Korean improved.

He studied hard for four years and still found time to continue playing tennis winning several trophies in both National Medical School Championships and among all Korean colleges and universities. Medical school in Korea was as grueling as medical school in America and filled with stories of failing classmates, tyrannical professors, exhaustion, and the occasional bright or humorous episode. Tom did have the opportunity to work with school medical missions in remote areas. This increased his desire to be a medical missionary, and fired his compassion for the poor. As graduation approached, Tom's father advised him to consider an internship and residency in the United States.

Tom Kim followed his father's advice and accepted an internship in Akron, Ohio. Prior to returning to the US, he had managed to find time to become engaged and married on April 20, 1974. His new bride stayed in Korea with her parents for six months while Tom completed the first phase of his training in Ohio. His internship included four rotations through Pediatrics, Ob/Gyn, Internal Medicine, and Surgery, that provided a firm foundation for his future free clinic primary care practice. A two year residency in Internal Medicine in Dayton, Ohio followed. The residency was at a VA Hospital and this work with veterans was a harbinger of future close ties with veterans of the Korean War. Tom then became Chief Resident at St. Agnes Hospital in Baltimore.

After five years training in America, he still felt called to return to Korea in some medical mission capacity. He had also decided that fighting cancer would be an important part of this venture. Needing two more years of training in hematology/oncology, Tom interviewed with the M.D. Anderson Center, Miami University, and UT Medical Center, finally picking the UT fellowship. So, in July 1979, the thirty-five year old Dr. Kim moved with his wife and baby girl to Knoxville, Tennessee.

Southern hospitality is not just a platitude. It played some part in the decision of this young family, living in what was still essentially a foreign culture, to plant roots in East Tennessee. Dr. Kim's wife liked the South, although not yet entirely comfortable in America. However, the natural kindness and generosity of the people, the conservatism of the area, and the birth of another child, combined to persuade the Kims to make this region their permanent home. A staff position at Baptist Hospital and association with a group practice followed the UT training. By 1983, Dr. Kim had moved into a solo practice, first on Sevier Avenue and later on Chapman Highway, becoming in his words, "My own boss."

This completes the story of how Dr. Tom Kim became a Knoxvillian. He survived two wars and escaped from communist tyranny. He endured long family separation and uncertainty, overcame the cultural shock of moving between Western and Oriental society multiple times, became an American physician, and finally settled in the hills of East Tennessee. Knowing this account helps to better understand how the Free Clinic moved from an idea to a reality in a few short months. Dr. Kim's drive, tenacity, and utter refusal to take no for an answer explain much about how the Free Clinic came to be.

The young man, who was not a quitter, became the middle aged doctor who would not give up when told something just couldn't be done. At the same time, Dr. Kim did not prosper in America without help.

Teachers, coaches, and friends helped him along the way. It was the same with the Free Clinic – he did not do it alone. However, without him there would be no Free Clinic in Knoxville. It will probably be the same with any other fast track clinic. Without a champion along the lines of Dr. Kim, it could take years to get the existing establishment to do it.

As a coda to this section, one might ask what happened to Dr. Kim's dream of a medical mission in Korea. It is still alive and currently focuses on a cancer hospice and retreat center overlooking the Sea of Japan where the poor can receive both the medical and spiritual care they so desperately need. Still, the Korean Hillbilly can also see the same need in his adopted home and the hospice may someday become a reality in the Smoky Mountains. That would be a fitting end to this story of East meets West.

THE SERMON

After the move to Chapman Highway, life became more settled for Dr. Tom Kim and his family. Golf replaced tennis, a solo medical practice replaced years of training, and a settled, but busy, family life replaced the nomad existence that had characterized life prior to Knoxville. Dr. Kim and Hwa had two growing children, daughter Kimberly and son Timothy. (Kimberly is now a pediatrician practicing at East Tennessee Children's Hospital and Tim works with Civicorps Schools, a non-profit organization in Oakland, California.) By the early nineties, Dr. Kim was living the American Dream. He was his own boss and had a great deal of freedom in how he would live his life.

Two notions remained a major part of his psyche. First was serving God and his fellow man. For him this seemed to mean Christian mission work. Second, was repaying the debt he felt he owed America. In his mind, US soldiers had saved his life during the Korean War and this country had welcomed him as a boy. He was grateful for these gifts. As he enjoyed a relatively comfortable life, he could not avoid the sense that he needed to do more. Establishing his practice as a going concern, providing a secure future for his family, and educating two children took most of his time and energy for several years. Still, his old desire for mission work was alive and well. The question was not if, but how?

For many years, mission work for Tom Kim had meant returning to Korea as a medical missionary. This had been the plan when he passed up the opportunity to attend medical school at Indiana University and returned to Korea for his basic medical education. It had been the plan when he trained for many years in America. After medical school, Dr. Kim had regained a command of the Korean language and this would increase his effectiveness in that country. There were many things that made him believe he would be the "perfect medical missionary to Korea."

How to accomplish this goal remained the question. He considered short-term mission work. Several organizations who wanted him to do short-term foreign mission work approached him. As with so many well-intended plans, the press of daily life stifled the possibility. He could not leave his private practice. So many people relied on him and, as a solo practitioner, covering his patient's need for the extended period even a short-term mission required was out of the question. Through a long process of prayer and soul searching, he arrived at a solution.

Dr. Kim decided to provide free medical care to the needy in Knoxville. He recognized it was not necessary to travel to a foreign land to do God's work. He would bloom where planted. The more he thought about this plan, the more he saw that it would fill many of the needs in his life. He could fulfill his desire to serve God and others. He could realize his particular compassion for the poor, first truly recognized during medical school field work in remote areas of Korea. And, as a bonus, it was a clear way of saying how grateful he was to America.

So, in 1993, Dr. Kim began what came to be known as The Free Medical Clinic of America. Although not formally chartered until 2005, the after-hours clinic had that name almost since the beginning. The clinic was initially a very informal affair. Dr. Kim just set aside some time to see patients in his office without charging them. He knew he could spend a few hours a week after regular office hours and perhaps get some volunteer nurses to help. Using his own office and some volunteer helpers meant that he did not need any outside help and he could make the medical services totally free.

He knew there was a need, but he wasn't sure of how to reach those who needed this particular assistance. A newspaper ad made sense so he called the local newspaper to place one. In the course of explaining what he wanted to do, the ad clerk realized there was a story here and suggested the newspaper do one. The newspaper promised a visit by a reporter and photographer within 72 hours and it was good to its word. On Saturday, June 26, 1993, an article appeared entitled, "Free Clinic set for working poor." The subtitle of the article was, "Doctor calls it longtime desire to repay America." These two short lines were the culmination of many years of thought, prayer, and planning. They also were the realization of important themes in Tom Kim's life – compassion for the poor, service of other people, and gratitude for his new life.

Dr. Kim chose July 1, 1993, as opening day for the after-hours clinic. He treated four patients that first day. The article also brought offers from volunteer nurses and the response gave Kim the option of rotating nurses. The "clinic" settled into a routine of opening at five in the afternoon Monday, Tuesday, Thursday, and Friday and staying open until six or seven in the evening, depending on the number of patients to be seen. A volunteer nurse would come to assist Dr. Kim as he saw patients after a full day in his own office. This was a very simple administrative operation that concentrated on delivering the medical skills of the doctor nurse team. This service was free and greatly appreciated. Often patients required medication and after writing a prescription Dr. Kim would try to find a drug sample furnished by pharmaceutical reps to give them. When necessary, he would also reach into his own pocket for the money to ensure that the patient got the needed medicine.

Early on, Dr. Kim was puzzled that more folks had not called upon his free clinic. The working poor, which were the target population, usually do not have many options for medical care and he knew the need was great. He reasoned that perhaps his target audience did not use the newspaper as their primary source of information and the clinic was relying on one article as the primary means of informing the public. Acting on this notion, he was able to arrange a local television interview with all three of the major affiliate stations in Knoxville. Dr. Kim had received a certificate of appreciation for the clinic from Congressman Jimmy Duncan and the stations were willing to cover that story. On December 14, 1993, a little over five months after opening, an account of the Free Clinic ran on Knoxville's six and eleven o'clock news shows. After that, spreading the word was not a problem. The clinic thrived, and on some days Dr. Kim saw more free care patients than his regular practice patients. By 2001 the clinic had completed several thousand appointments. Surely Dr. Kim could slow down and rest a little. Of course not!

Driven to do more, he looked for further opportunities to serve the poor with his medical skills. In January 2002, he broadened this work by extending the Free Medical Clinic of America to Briceville, Tennessee and seeing patients every Wednesday. (Who wants to play golf every Wednesday anyway?) Briceville is in Anderson County and is in the heart of coal mining country. But, the mines closed and the community suffered. Again the needs were great and Dr. Kim began seeing patients in a donated building. Patients could not make an appointment because there was no phone. They just knew that, if you were sick and needed care, show up on Wednesday morning and Dr. Kim would help you.

From that January, both the free clinics in Dr. Kim's office and at the Briceville location continued to see patients at no charge. Dr. Kim was doing all he could to minister to his neighbors and bring some relief to the working poor of the area. He had very little free time because the free clinic work came after-hours. He believed that this was the way to do mission work. To some degree, he was following the example of the Apostle Paul who was always willing to work while his real mission in life was to spread the gospel. Dr. Kim had struggled with this concept and had reached the conclusion that the best way was to "use your own time and your own money."

With a few volunteer nurses, Dr. Kim was able to see a significant number of patients in his after-hours clinic and at Briceville. It was always clear that demand for these services far outstripped supply. Emergency rooms, doctor locator services, hospitals, health departments, and other charitable clinics referred patients to Dr. Kim. Distance didn't seem to matter. Patients came from throughout East Tennessee as news about his work spread, often simply by word of mouth. Typically, Dr. Kim did not keep statistics. He really couldn't report how many patients he had seen or the value of the free medical care he delivered. Counting "nickels and noses" did not interest him. He was content to say, "If I help one person a day, I'm more than happy."

Dr. Kim had reason to be happy. As noted, he had already helped thousands of individuals with free medical care possibly worth of millions of dollars. And, he did it his way with no muss and no fuss. The clinic was not incorporated. He did not answer to a board. He spent no time raising funds and over a twelve year period volunteer nurses had appeared when needed. He was free to concentrate on helping the working poor with his medical skills and that he did in full measure. Perhaps it was time to say I've done my part and let someone else put on the mantle of self-supporting medical missionary to East Tennessee. Besides, he was over sixty years old and how much sacrifice is enough.

As so often happens when one asks these "life" questions, the answer came loud and clear. As a life long Presbyterian, Dr. Kim and his family were attending a local Presbyterian church. The church supported many missions and individual missionaries. The senior pastor often preached sermons that stressed Christian service. In early 2005, Dr. Kim heard such a sermon on the subject of "Love Your Neighbor." To Dr. Kim, the gist of the sermon was that, if you truly loved your neighbor, you could not give too much. There were no limits on God's love, so why should there be limits on our love for others.

This message quickly became a part of Tom Kim's consciousness. He processed the concept and considered what it could mean. Was he to simply give more time? He was devoting well over fifteen hours a week to his free clinic work. Was he to increase that to thirty hours? It was clear there were physical limits to what he could do or be expected to do. How would this desire to love his neighbor in the way implied by that sermon work its way out in his life? In a pattern established early in his life, Dr. Kim quickly came to a decision.

For Kim, a quick decision does not mean a cavalier or casual decision. It does not mean a decision without thought or research. It does not mean a decision without prayer and searching for God's leading. It means that when the answer is loud and clear, you act. When the train pulls out of the station for South Korea, you should be on it because there may not be another one. You don't wait to pack your bags, you act. His medical training had reinforced this principle. Sometimes you must act with less than perfect knowledge, and often it is better to do "something" than to do "nothing."

So as the sermon rebounded in his mind, Dr. Kim came to what to him was an unexpected conclusion. He could not do it all by himself. There was a limit to what "Dr. Kim's Free Clinic" could do. There were only marginal increases that the current after-hours clinic could support. He reasoned that, if he was willing to give several hours a week helping the working poor, surely other doctors in the community would be willing to do the same. They would not have to commit to fifteen hours a week. If several physicians would give just a few hours a month, then he could organize something to deliver this care on a regular and expanded basis. What do you call something organized to deliver medical care on a regular basis that does not charge for the service? Obviously, you call it a free clinic.

Thus, for Dr. Kim, the fruit of the sermon preached on Sunday, January 23, 2005, became a free clinic. Dr. Kim believed Knoxville needed a new free clinic. Exactly what this meant was not yet clear, but there was enough clarity to start moving. Another train was leaving the station and it was time to jump on board.

So what if you don't know exactly where the train is headed as long as it is clear it is going in the right direction. Tom Kim had moved from the idea of "Dr. Kim's Free Clinic," of which he was chief cook and bottle washer as well as the attending physician, to a "Community Free Clinic" where he was only one of many serving in various capacities.

The notion of a community free clinic was uncharted territory for Dr. Kim. The thought of expanding his after-hours clinic to a full-time clinic was daunting in many ways. For one thing, a clinic of this scope could not be no muss and no fuss. There was so much to do in terms of the administrative, legal, and medical concerns. A community free clinic was certainly more than one person could handle. This would require a more formal organization. Governance and operation of the organization would require that many hearts, hands, and heads be involved.

A description of the journey from the rudimentary idea of a community free clinic to the current Free Clinic in Knoxville, Tennessee follows. Its beginning was one sermon that fired a passion in one man to love his neighbor through a free medical clinic. It is an account of the steps that were necessary to move from a vision to reality on the ground in a few short months.

LEAP OF FAITH

Dr. Kim now had a plan. A free clinic open many hours a week would replace his limited after-hours clinic. It would be entirely free to the working, uninsured. It would rely on volunteers. It would be, as much as possible, a simple and lean operation. It would be an extension of his own approach to loving his neighbor, which was just doing something for them. If you have a skill, make it available to those who need it. If you have some free time, use it to help others. If you have some extra cash, donate it to a worthy cause, preferably one in which you are willing to invest your time as well. It seemed like a simple plan. Surely the community would be willing to support such an approach.

He believed that, when given a clear opportunity to serve, most folks would respond to the call. He had not had any problem finding volunteer nurses to help him with the initial free clinic venture. He had received many calls and offers to help. As he looked forward to an expanded free clinic, he assumed he could count on the same response. As a practicing physician, he was in daily contact with nurses and casual conversation spread the word about the intended need. He had many retired nurses among his friends who were looking for a few hours service a week to keep them busy. As a staff member, he had met and become friends with many hospital volunteers. Many had said they were willing to answer phones, make appointments, register patients, and perform the myriad of tasks he knew a larger clinic would entail. It was reasonable for Dr. Kim to believe that all he had to do was let the community know about his plan and willing workers would appear.

Dr. Kim had the basic plan in his head, but as he shared it with others he had to face reality. Not everyone shared his enthusiasm for either helping the needy or doing it in exactly the way that he outlined. He often had roadblocks, real or imagined, thrown in the path. To be fair to Knoxville, the objections were ones that most community assistance projects and programs face no matter where located. For most individuals the objections represented an acceptance of reality more than a reluctance to commit or contribute to the idea of community service. Any group that starts a community project should expect these and similar concerns. Clinic planners should also bear in mind that a medical clinic has some particular concerns.

Jack McConnell and the Volunteers in Medicine (VIM) Clinic on Hilton Head Island were cited in the Prologue. VIM experienced every obstacle faced by Dr. Kim in the opening of their clinic. The solution to each objection was not necessarily exactly the same, but the overall path to opening a clinic was certainly comparable. When Tom Kim asked what others thought about his plan for a community free clinic, he found that many people had doubts about the feasibility of such an undertaking. Individuals tended to phrase these anxieties as a question. Six questions were most often asked.

First, medical professionals usually asked the threshold question, "Can't I get sued for doing this?" Doctors and nurses don't want any exposure to malpractice claims beyond what they face in their regular jobs. No matter how great the need or how motivated to serve, most medical professionals feel absolutely obligated to make this their first consideration. Whenever they think about using their medical skills outside the confines of their regular employment, they must protect themselves. Good Samaritan laws notwithstanding, they sense that when they venture beyond their daily routine they somehow increase their exposure. This is a pervasive concern for all medical professionals.

There is some interesting anecdotal data that suggests that many doctors and nurses who routinely participate in foreign mission trips, whether religious or secular sponsored, do so because they believe they serve with virtually no risk of malpractice claims. There is usually some underlying indemnification and jurisdictional factors that make a lawsuit appear very unlikely. The point appears to be some doctors and nurses motivated to serve as volunteers believe service in their local communities may be inherently more risky than overseas service.

Medical professionals who have been in lawsuits frequently report that a successful outcome is immaterial. Suits settled for essentially nuisance value by the insurance companies are still a part of their professional history. Being held completely blameless is no comfort. The time lost in depositions, trial preparation, and in court is not balanced by the most favorable verdict.

This is not a discourse on current laws or any aspect of medical practice. It is simply to point out that, when asking medical professionals to volunteer their services; their first question will usually be some form of "what is my malpractice exposure?" If there is not an adequate answer to that question, there will be little more discussion. Many are willing to donate their time and medical skills, but they must have a clear answer to this major concern. Any community free clinic that intends to rely on medical volunteers must address this issue in detail and to the satisfaction of the potential volunteers.

Closely related is the question of licensing. For example, at Hilton Head, the volunteer pool was virtually all retired doctors, many from states other than South Carolina. They did not want to take an exam or pay high fees for a license in their retirement state. Dr. McConnell overcame this major hurdle through some creative lobbying and politicking with the South Carolina Legislature. This issue was not a problem in Knoxville because virtually all medical professionals contacted had Tennessee licenses and practiced in the community, but it can be a major concern in other situations.

The second question was, "Shouldn't government take care of that?" There is a reasonable expectation among Americans that the government will take care of the basic necessities of those who need help such as health care. While far from reality, this notion is understandable when one considers the plethora of agencies, federal, state, and local, that most Americans recognize by their familiar acronyms. Many Americans instinctively think of Medicare, Medicaid, SCHIPS, Department of Health, DCS, and a host of others in the alphabet soup of contemporary agencies delivering health care. It is not unreasonable that the first reaction of many people is often that the need is, or should be, covered by some government entity.

In Knoxville, some potential support groups and individuals contacted seemed to share this view to varying degrees. The notion that health care is a government function was wide spread and was a prominent response among both medical and non-medical groups. Individuals frequently used "It's not our job" as a rationale for not pursuing a free clinic.

Frankly, a few folks had a rather bleak outlook that seemed to center on the feeling that, "I pay taxes and a lot of that money goes to the poor." It was also amazing to find that some people felt that inadequate access to medical care was a failure on the part of the individual. Lack of a willingness to work and poor life style choices were cited as the proximate causes of their need. "Some people let that happen and they must suffer the consequences. If government wants to bail them out I can't do much about that, but I won't support their poor choices." When looking for clinic support, planners must occasionally expect similar uninformed and unsympathetic views.

When making these arguments, there is always a kernel of truth that can make them sound sensible. As noted there are many ways that government delivers health care to its citizens. Most notably, the elderly, the young, the very poor, and some special cases, such as renal failure, usually do have government coverage when needed. Generally, the well-off, the well-employed, and the lucky have access to private insurance. However, those who make too much to qualify for public assistance and too little to afford their own care have very few options. Many must choose between feeding their family and medical care, so they opt for food. With the current trend of employers either not offering health insurance or "cost shifting" to employees, even full employment does not guarantee minimum medical needs are met. A permanent medically under-served element is a reality in America.

Just in the Knoxville area, the estimated number of uninsured individuals has been reported as high as eighty thousand. That means they do not have coverage under any of the government programs or private insurers. The hard truth is that there is a tremendous health care gap to slip through and many do. Thousands of hard working folk, who pay taxes and contribute in many other ways to their community, do not have ready access to public or private

Five Fingers

---

health care. When soliciting support for a community free clinic, expect to hear the objection that providing health care is a government responsibility. Many people honestly believe that government is doing an adequate job of ensuring health care for all who need it. Be prepared to present the facts that show this is simply not the case.

The third question encountered was, "Don't others already do that?" There are many individuals and groups that do recognize that government can not meet all the current needs. TV, radio, the internet, and print media often cite national uninsured statistics, and include what is being done in the non-governmental sector to address these needs. Again, Knoxville presents a typical example of why there can be the erroneous assumption that non-profits and other organizations are meeting any need not covered by government agencies.

There are many different groups providing some form of reduced charge or free medical care in the Knoxville area. To name a few: Volunteer Rescue Ministries, Knoxville Area Rescue Ministries, The Salvation Army, InterFaith Clinic, Remote Area Medical, and Knoxville Area Project Access all offer some form of medical care. These well-established groups engage in fund raising as a matter of course that often makes them high profile organizations. Many local people know and respect the work they do.

In addition, broader service organizations such as United Way are perceived as supporting the medically under-served. Knoxville also has a number of quiet philanthropists who support caring for those with medical needs. They generally avoid publicity and recognition, but many know of their work and generosity. Again, the point is that the notion that others are already seeing to the medical needs of the uninsured may seem reasonable. The many examples of medical service organizations cited in this section would make many think that the supply side of health care, at least in Knoxville, is adequate.

Nothing could be further from reality. In this area, as in most of the country, the demand for uninsured health care far outstrips supply. Any number of needs assessments, surveys, and statistical analysis make it clear that there are not anywhere near adequate resources. A commonsense analysis also verifies the gap. Existing facilities have long waiting lists. Depending on the service required, a patient might wait weeks for an appointment or be told that the particular service they need is just not available. If a new facility opens or a new service offered at an existing one, it can expect a large number of requests for service.

The objection that others are already filling the gap is rarely mean spirited. It is commonly a sincere argument that makes two points. One is that there are existing non-governmental organizations helping the uninsured. Second is that support of one is made at the expense of the others. The pie is only so big and when a new organization receives support it simply means some others must receive less. This is the overworked "zero sum game." This is a logical argument, particularly when it comes from someone who is already generously supporting other projects and programs.

A part of the answer to this argument lies in the fact that specifically in Knoxville, and in general throughout the country, uninsured health care providers cooperate closely and coordinate their efforts. For example, the Free Clinic has limited specialty services and refers these cases to other providers. It concentrates on primary care and basic diagnostic services that relieve the burden on other clinics that offer more comprehensive services. Each provider plays an important role in meeting the needs of the uninsured.

This cooperation facilitates a division of labor and economy of scale. Since primary care clinics do fewer things, have no specialists, and limited equipment, they usually deliver care at a lower cost. Having and supporting multiple sources of health care makes the overall delivery more efficient. So, rather than diluting the effect of health care spending, adding and supporting additional resources may actually improve efficiency, giving more bang to each buck. The need for these approaches will continue as long as the demand for free health care exceeds the supply.

"Why do you want to start a clinic, don't established institutions do things like that?" Asking this fourth question was really asking, "Don't our hospitals take care of that?" A hospital normally requires a certificate of need to open or continue to operate. Certain obligations go along with that franchise. Indigent care, emergency rooms, and community outreach may be among the requirements. Many perceive these things as providing a floor or safety net for the uninsured. That no one can be turned away from an emergency room is a prevailing notion in many discussions of uninsured health care. It also may be a concept often more honored in the breach than in the practice.

Closing emergency rooms, limiting services, and transferring patients are all examples of how hospitals could deal with the demands of the uninsured on their emergency facilities. In reality, emergency rooms are not an adequate safety net for the uninsured. The uninsured may not turn to an emergency room until their condition is extremely serious or painful. Then the cost of restorative care versus preventative care becomes clear. Through no fault of their own, hospitals are an expensive and inefficient means of delivering health care to the uninsured.

Losses in the emergency room may be one of the sources of the financial shortfall for hospitals. When uninsured individuals seek treatment at ERs, some routinely, most of the costs are uncollectable and written-off. Not all community free clinic visits would otherwise result in an ER treatment; but, if they did, the cost is usually in the millions of dollars. One free clinic in Chattanooga, Tennessee estimates it has saved the community sixteen million dollars in ER costs in less than five years. The similar sized Free Clinic in Knoxville claims a more modest eight million dollars for the same period.

The warning is that when seeking support for a community free clinic initiative, be prepared for the contention that hospitals cover that need as a provider of last resort. What is strange is that free clinic sponsors may find that local hospitals have mixed feelings about opening clinics. For example, in Hilton Head the local hospital first opposed the clinic, but eventually became a supporter. In other cases, hospitals that see a new free clinic as a means of relieving pressure on their ER can be enthusiastic supporters from the start. Be prepared for either eventuality.

The fifth question was, "How long is starting a clinic going to take?" Again, the not so hidden implication is you might be able to do it, but it will take a very long time. Starting a community free clinic can take a long time. There will be plenty of hurdles to overcome and the planners can't handle them in a slipshod manner. It may take a while, but the Knoxville Free Clinic became a reality in about six months. Others may take years from concept to fruition. Speed is not the issue. Will is the issue. When a critical mass of folks see a need and have the will to see it met, they will find a solution. Be prepared for the question of how long, but do not let it drive your efforts. "Yes, it's going to take some time, so let's get started," may be the best answer to this question.

The sixth and final question is not unique to health care or any particular charitable endeavor. Without being too clever, this can be phrased as, "Don't you know I already gave at the office?" This can be an expected response when soliciting financial or other support for any new venture. In truth, many of the individuals or organizations solicited will have already given very generously to many different causes. A few are simply avoiding you. Most are sincere, or at least believe in their hearts they have done their part. Giving to the United Way clears the deck emotionally for many Americans.

When you approach potential supporters, you must have a story to tell. That story will vary in every locale. Be sure you know that story and articulate it well. Show how providing health care will solve other problems as well. Facts and figures are always important, but putting a human face on your story seems to be more important. Providing health care to the uninsured is one area where the human element is not hard to find. Every case of a diabetic father going without medication to feed his family is an intensely human narrative. A single mother working two or three jobs without any health insurance carries its own weight. Again, be prepared for the claim that we have already given as a last line of resistance.

In summary, when Tom Kim shopped around his idea of opening a community free clinic, he heard six standard objections. Concisely stated they are: 1) I cannot risk being sued, 2) Government should do that, 3) Other groups do that, 4) Hospitals already do that, 5) It will take too long, and 6) I give my support elsewhere. These were not the only concerns about supporting the new clinic, but they cover the most important areas.

Hearing these rejections of his plan was discouraging and that is why the next step for Tom Kim became a Leap of Faith. Tom listened to those who said it couldn't be done, but he concluded that it could. All it would take is the faith to start the ball rolling. The plan would pick up speed on its own and he committed to overcome this initial inertia to a new clinic.

With so much against his plan, it would be a miracle if he could accomplish it. In spite of this and acting on faith, Dr. Tom Kim ignored the naysayers and scheduled a public meeting to test support. He announced it and, again, the local newspaper supported Tom with an article explaining in detail his concern and general plan. The paper reported the purpose of the "forum in West Knoxville [is] to address the health needs of the working poor." "[H]ealth professionals of all types ... as well as the general public" were invited to attend. Tom was fully committed and he was now ready to go public with his plan.

THE MEETING

It sometimes seems that in America if you don't really want to do something but want to appear busy, you schedule a meeting. This notion may come from sources such as the *Dilbert* cartoon series where meetings are portrayed as ineffective at best. The meeting that Dr. Kim called was not immune from this criticism, but nothing could be further from the truth. He did not schedule the meeting to appear busy, pass off the workload, or spread responsibility. As stated, he did it as a leap of faith because he trusted that support for a new clinic would materialize.

Tom Kim had faith that others shared his compassion for the poor and would see that providing health care was a tangible, worthwhile ministry. He was certain that many individuals would respond to a call to expand his work with the uninsured. He felt his after-hours clinic could rapidly expand into a more comprehensive community clinic. He announced his plan and was certain that all he needed to do was to initially get things moving. Since this narrative is to serve in some part as a road map to opening future clinics, the meeting will be described in detail.

Dr. Kim announced the meeting in an article on February 18, 2005, in the local newspaper. The Knoxville News-Sentinel had provided wonderful coverage of Kim's previous efforts to help the working uninsured. They had done several articles over the years, beginning with the initial article triggered by his inquiry about placing a classified ad. The support of local media is essential to moving along any effort to start a community clinic. In this regard, Kim was fortunate to have the support of not only the local newspaper, but television also. A positive relationship with all local media must be established and nurtured, and this must be done when the clinic is only a dream in the mind of the founding champions.

The newspaper article was in the Friday paper. Friday is the day chosen by the paper to highlight local health care coverage, so it was a logical choice. Saturday at 10:00 a.m. – the very next day, were the time and date of the meeting. The article served as the first, final, and official notice of the meeting, but Dr. Kim had worked the phone and his personal contacts for many days prior to the article. Again, Kim kept in mind the lesson previously learned that not everybody gets their news from the print media today, and used TV and other forms of communication as well. However, the newspaper article remains the best record of the meeting and will be quoted extensively.

The article was titled, "Doctor reaches out to aid working poor," and subtitled, "Forum planned to seek help in founding clinic to offer free health care."

It quickly summarized Dr. Kim's past efforts in his office and asked "other health professionals to lend a helping hand." The goal of the meeting was to gather support for "a free clinic for those who are unable to pay for a trip to a doctor." The appeal was not to just medical professionals, but to the community at large. "[Kim] is inviting health professionals of all types as well as the general public."

Kim stressed that the clinic would be all volunteers, "no one is going to be paid, so there will be no overhead." "Doctors and nurses, lawyers and pharmacists, they can all come help with this." Children were also invited to the meeting and parents asked to bring them. "By having the children join in the discussion, we will be showing our love and concern for them, while teaching them to become our future community leaders." There were high expectations for the meeting.

The meeting was to take place in the Family Life Center of Cedar Springs Presbyterian Church in West Knoxville. Kim had asked if he could use the church's small chapel to host a meeting. Naturally, he was asked for details. Kim explained his plan and was offered the larger fellowship hall and other church support for the forum.

A Sunday, February 20, 2005, article in the News-Sentinel reports on the results of the Saturday meeting. The headline of, "Crowd turns out for health-care forum," marks the tenor of the piece. Since a reporter with some experience covering local medical issues wrote the article, it marks the meeting as a success in terms of the numbers responding to the invitation and the meeting outcomes.

The subtitle, "Number of concerned citizens at discussion surprises Knox doctor," reinforces this point. The turnout impressed Dr. Kim and boded well for the future clinic. A "cross section of the concerned" attended and showed interest in helping make Kim's dream a reality. Kim is quoted as saying, "I was surprised by the number of people who showed support. It was fantastic. Everyone is really concerned. We had politicians, pharmacists, retired people, nurses– just a wide variety of people there."

The newspaper article did not report actual attendance, but Kim recalls the medical professional attendance as: seven physicians, a podiatrist, two dentists, three nurses, two pharmacists, and seven administrative health professionals. Particularly encouraging was the number of non-medical personnel who attended, which included at least one attorney and two ministers. Individuals simply interested in improving their community far outnumbered the medical professionals. Kim knew from experience that folks willing to fill the volunteer administrative positions required to operate a full-time clinic would be critical to its success. In all about 200 people showed up for the meeting.

The agenda included several short presentations with well-known TV personality Bill Williams serving as master of ceremonies. Kim covered the now familiar estimate of fifty million Americans without health insurance. His point was to draw attention to the overwhelming need. More to his point, he moved to a discussion of the impending cuts in TennCare, Tennessee's Medicaid program. Plans for changes in eligibility announced recently indicated substantial cuts in the number of Tennesseeans covered would be made.

In this regard, Dr. Kim's timing was fortuitous because most Tennessee communities were drafting plans to deal with a significant increase in the uninsured. A new community free clinic in Knoxville, although it would be the new kid on the block, would certainly be welcome. In its first year of operation, forty-three percent of Free Clinic patients self-reported losing TennCare coverage. Estimates are that about 200,000 individuals lost their coverage on or near August 31, 2005, one month after the opening of the Free Clinic.

Those in attendance had the opportunity to "sign up" as volunteers in various capacities. The Foundation staff present collected names, phone numbers, and e-mail addresses for anyone willing to help with the clinic. This sign-up list provided a working roster of potential volunteers and clinic staff. Dr. Kim left the forum feeling that the hardest part of bringing the clinic into being was behind him. He had shared his vision and the response was great.

Buried in the article is a sentence that "Kim is also planning to go to Sri Lanka and help tsunami victims in upcoming months." This proved, in many ways, to be the operative outcome of the meeting. Dr. Kim did go to Sri Lanka spending almost two weeks, from early to mid March on the trip. Kim had left with the impression, or at least the hope, that on his return the planning for the new clinic would be well under way and substantial milestones accomplished. Chief among these was a place to house the clinic. He had listed finding a suitable place for the clinic the major requirement. The February 18 article announcing the meeting had obliquely referred to this necessity. Kim had said, "There won't be any overhead." "All we need is the building and maintenance."

When Kim returned from his tsunami mission work, he found that very little had been accomplished in his absence. There certainly was no building located as the home of the clinic. No one had taken this responsibility and addressed it while he was away. Had the concern and support evinced in the February 19 meeting evaporated? It appeared to him that it had. Tom Kim, the athlete, workaholic, and focused advocate of a new Knoxville community free clinic was, in a word, discouraged. Why didn't others share the same drive and determination to succeed at any cost that was such a large part of his character? Why wasn't more accomplished while he was away serving in another corner of this needy world?

A couple of lessons were learned from the circumstances detailed above. These lessons are extremely important to any group that is considering starting a clinic. The first is that no two individuals see any situation in exactly the same light. The folks who attended the Saturday morning meeting saw themselves as committed and concerned. They saw their commitment as high. Truth be told, Kim saw it as low.

There was little to show for two weeks, not because no one cared, but because no specific individual felt empowered and responsible for moving things along. Most folks probably thought things were going pretty well. They could see progress just in airing the concerns and discussing solutions in general terms. This may be fine if your time line is two years to open a clinic. Dr. Kim valued and appreciated this view, he just did not agree with it. Where others saw progress and potential, he saw wasted time and opportunity. Things couldn't move too fast for him; and, in his mind, they were moving far too slowly.

Individuals or groups supporting the effort will always view the pace of work and progress very differently. Like Goldilocks, some will say too fast, some will say too slow, and a very few will say just right. Consider all evaluations and honor the contributions of all. Many of the original meeting attendees have become some of the strongest supporters of the Free Clinic. If Dr. Kim had succumbed to the initial wave of discouragement he felt upon his return and reacted rashly, he might have lost some of the clinic's greatest allies.

The second lesson learned follows directly from the first. The lost time was not due to a lack of commitment per se, but rather to the lack of a champion. Every organization successfully involved in opening a community free clinic has noted the absolute need for a champion. The champion is someone who organizes, motivates, inspires, and facilitates every aspect of the project. The champion can be an individual, but the most effective ones are small groups of like minded individuals. A civic club subcommittee, a small Sunday School Class, or a group of neighbors can become free clinic champions.

The group can not be too large, because it quickly becomes ineffective. It can be one man, as in the case of Dr. Kim, but the danger here is that the champion becomes spread too thin. Dr. Kim was the only one who knew the master plan and when he left the scene for a short time, progress came to a standstill. The clinic champion is a combination taskmaster, overseer, cheerleader, psychiatrist, and hand-holder. He must guide clinic planners through demanding times. When the champion is not pushing the group, motivation may wane and progress slow. Champions can expect to do little else once they set out on the path to a free clinic. They must understand and commit to the arduous nature of the task.

Along with these lessons, the importance of sympathetic media must be stressed. The Free Clinic was blessed to have the enthusiastic support of the local media, to include print, television and radio. All along the way, Dr. Kim and the clinic planners strove to provide the media with the best possible information and put a human face on it.

Putting a human face on that information means explaining it in terms of real cases. One example is a diabetic patient who regularly comes to the clinic for medication and a checkup. The patient says that before she found the clinic she simply went without any treatment. At first, she needed help to pay for medication. When the story ends that one day she proudly states that she feels so much better she is working enough to get a little ahead. She then pulls a crumbled five dollar bill from her pocket and insists that the clinic accept it. That story has a human face. It is hard to make a connection until something helps an outsider to see the individuals behind the numbers.

Dr. Kim went into the February meeting as a leap of faith. He didn't listen to those who said it couldn't be done. He called for a community forum and the turnout and initial reaction surprised and gratified him. Then he had to face the reality that one meeting was not enough to overcome inertia. Opening a new clinic would require much more work. To say that the February meeting was all lip service is both untrue and unfair. The meeting touched many hearts and prepared individuals to volunteer later. The publicity alone was worth the effort because it prepared the community to accept the clinic when it debuted in August. While it did not meet the high expectations of Dr. Kim, it was an important step to the present day Free Clinic. The story continues as Tom Kim, the old wrestler, begins to adopt a more aggressive attitude.

A CHANGE OF PACE

When Dr. Kim returned from Sri Lanka, he faced a very low point. During the mission trip he had suffered from excruciating back pain that had left him physically and mentally exhausted. (He would finally require surgery for the condition in the summer of 2008.) He not only was tired, but also had to deal with what he saw as a lack of progress on the clinic. Tom Kim dreams big and it would be difficult for any progress toward a new clinic to meet his expectations. The slow movement during his absence disappointed him to say the least. With his physical condition clearly playing a role, he had mixed feelings about the future of the clinic.

However, Tom Kim is nothing if not an optimist. He has often said that as one awakes in the morning and smells that first, fresh cup of coffee, the world looks a lot different. The body can refresh itself with a good night's sleep and the mind can refocus on the task at hand. "They who wait upon the Lord shall renew their strength," is more than a passage from

Five Fingers

the Bible to him. It is a way of life that expects some discouragement, but must not allow it to be a reason to quit. It took a couple of days to recover, but he soon was ready to continue his mission.

At this point any form of encouragement would be welcome. The first exciting, example of support came from close at home. His wife Hwa suggested that he simply use the now vacant portion of his own office building as the home of the new clinic. Dr. Kim was pleased and a little chagrined that he had not thought of this earlier. He had often scouted possible locations throughout town, but had never found an appropriate site. Perhaps there was a reason he had not returned home to a done deal for clinic space.

The facility had most recently been a dentist's office and this offered some real advantages. It was close at hand which meant Kim could continue his private practice for sometime and still be readily available during clinic operating hours. There would be a ready made initial clientele from the patients currently treated in the after-hours clinic in his regular office. The clinic would be in an area that clearly needed such a clinic. It was close to the hospital where Kim had many friends and professional associates. As a dentist's office, although it would require some remodeling, it could be easily and quickly adapted to the needs of a medical clinic.

This turn of events not only encouraged Kim, but also suggested to him that it might be the time for more direct action than reflection. Twice, he had given a larger group the chance to take the lead. His first attempt had been to persuade the broad medical and community groups in Knoxville to support the plan. As explained, this met with well reasoned, but firm "nos." The second was to narrow his target audience to the folks turning out on a Saturday morning. They had expressed support by attending his February meeting. There was some encouragement from this group, but little tangible progress. This time he would be willing to do more of the work himself.

Dr. Kim never assumed he was the only person who cared about or could start a community clinic. Free or low charge clinics for the working poor already existed in Knoxville and in other towns and cities. He knew he needed help and lots of it. He wanted help, support, and advice and believed many individuals would assist when given a clear appeal for specific help. So, Tom Kim set out on a path best described as not asking, "What do you think about starting a clinic," to one of asking, "Will you do this to start a new clinic?"

This change in approach and philosophy is not a small one. It became the essence of getting things done to move the clinic along. In a gentle way, Kim wanted to simply ask, "Will you do this [task] for me?" He already knew the arguments against a new clinic and the reasons to go slowly. He now wanted to put the clinic on a fast track. If a group waits for things to be absolutely perfect, they might have to wait forever. Fast tracking means to take some risk.

Kim had committed to doing whatever it took to open a new clinic. He was going to take risks. He was going to work with smaller groups or individuals. He had learned many times over that a "no" to a request for help was not the worse thing that could happen. Not to ask was to assure a negative. Adopting the attitude that "they can only say no," gave him increased energy and motivation to ask for what might seem the impossible.

With this new approach and renewed energy, Kim began to layout the most important things to accomplish. A home for the clinic remained first on his list. The plan to use the vacant dentist's office next door made good sense, but would include remodeling. Remodeling meant money. Dr. Kim had returned so much in free care to the community in his years of private practice that he could not manage this expense by himself. He would need help. He first went to the executive management of Baptist Health System in Knoxville, because he knew the staff so well.

Baptist enthusiastically welcomed him and his plan. After Tom outlined both the physical expansion and the increased operating hours and patient capacity, Baptist Health System President & CEO referred him with a solid recommendation to The Baptist Health System Foundation. The Foundation was the philanthropic arm of the system and well experienced in these projects. Foundation President & CEO, Terry Morgan quickly gave the go ahead to start the renovation and began work on the many other tasks necessary to open a new clinic. The Foundation knew what they were doing because community outreach was a large part of their mission of community service. They had worked with other clinics and had a great deal of advice and practical experience to offer. The importance of the Baptist Health System Foundation to the Free Clinic cannot be overstated. Dr. Kim was the champion of the clinic, but The Foundation staff members were the key operators and partners. They gave substance to the vision and dreams of Dr. Kim. He pushed and they delivered.

It was at this time that the term "Nike Clinic" was coined. The Foundation staff members quickly became accustomed to Dr. Kim saying, "Don't worry about that, let's just do something." They naturally associated this attitude with the popular Nike Shoe Company slogan *Just Do It*, thus the sobriquet "Nike Clinic." Action was the primary requirement. If some things needed to be refined later, that was OK. Just get it done! When people advocate that others get out of their comfort zone, they must be talking about something like Dr. Kim's approach to opening the clinic. He had tried other approaches and now it was time to just act. The Foundation staffers were the first to fully understand the extent to which Tom Kim applied this operating principle and came up with an appropriate nickname.

The phrase "Tolerance for Ambiguity" is used by many authors and commentators. It was certainly a requirement in the flurry of activity surrounding the opening of the Free Clinic. Major decisions, such as how to make patient appointments, were tabled with the assertion, "it'll work itself out." If you wanted exact procedures in detail, you wouldn't get them in the run-up to the clinic opening. In Kim's mind, ambiguity could be tolerated for the greater good of simply having a clinic.

The remodeling work on the clinic was underway and The Foundation was tackling as much detail as it could. This left Dr. Kim relatively free to concentrate on those tasks that required his particular skills. His foremost task was lining up volunteer doctors and nurses to work in the clinic. As a medical professional he was in constant contact with doctors and nurses, and he was not bashful about asking for help. Although twisting an arm is an illegal move in wrestling, Dr. Kim was not afraid to apply a little torque when soliciting volunteers for the future clinic. More than one physician has executed a smart about face when he saw Dr. Tom Kim coming down a Baptist Hospital hallway in the spring and early summer of 2005.

On a more serious note, Dr. Kim knew from personal experience how valuable free time was to any medical professional. He knew he was asking a lot when he asked for "three or four hours a week," or "a couple of afternoons a month." He tried to emphasize the need and the positive impact it could have. He was presenting an opportunity to love your neighbor and that was a compelling argument to most of his contacts. He worked the hallways, the lounges, and the telephone to ensure the medical personnel would be there to staff the new clinic to be housed in the new facility.

Securing commitments from doctors was basically a one on one activity for Dr. Kim. Once a doctor responded to the call, it was important to find a time slot that would fit his or her schedule. This required some negotiation to fit the needs of the clinic with the needs of the volunteer. Due to its limited size, the clinic functions most efficiently with only one physician treating patients at a time. In some cases this made scheduling harder, such as when two doctors could work on a particular afternoon. Certain time periods were hard to fill, and others would have more than one potential volunteer. Part of the appeal of a large pool of volunteer doctors was that no one doctor would have to make an excessive contribution of time. Kim worked hard to obtain as many doctors as possible and to accommodate their individual schedules.

The clinic would obviously be a primary care facility and Dr. Kim knew well from his years of experience what to expect. This meant that "generalists," (i.e., general practitioners, family medicine, internists, etc.) would be best suited to meet the needs of free clinic patients. The clinic welcomed specialists, but generally they did not expect to "specialize" at the clinic. There would be exceptions to this rule, with the most notable being OB/GYN. Volunteer specialists would generally take referrals from the clinic and treat them in their own offices. The success of Dr. Kim's efforts is demonstrated by the fact that the first Free Clinic brochure, published prior to opening, listed fifty-seven MDs "committed to serve."

Dr. Kim also set about securing laboratory services for the clinic. He had a long established relationship with Laboratory Corporation of American, headquartered in Louisville Kentucky, to furnish all the equipment and supplies, pickup, testing, and reporting services for the numerous blood tests expected. Lab

Corp was an invaluable partner from the start. The number of tests required exceeded expectations, but Lab Corp met the demands and has been a stalwart in-kind service donor from the very beginning.

In all the previous years of delivering free medical care, Dr. Kim had personally funded all costs. The new community free clinic would extend the number of patients treated beyond his ability to continue this individual funding. As much as he disliked the task, he would have to devote some time to fund raising. Here again The Foundation had a ready made solution. The Foundation established an account to receive and disburse funds for the clinic. Donors were able to make donations to The Foundation in the clinic's name and receive full tax deductibility. This relieved Dr. Kim and the clinic of a number of burdensome accounting and administrative tasks.

This was an important service and operating principle for the clinic in its first days. It meant the clinic could function with the highest business, legal, and ethical standards with virtually no internal resources. This greatly eased the pressure on Kim and his supporters. The clinic might never have opened without The Foundation. The point to be made here is that during the planning and preparation phase The Foundation allowed Dr. Kim to focus his attention on those things he could do best.

A final example of the help that Kim sought and received during this time frame was from drug company representatives. Drug reps were eager to make the allowed contributions to a clinic that had already garnered a great deal of favorable publicity.

They donated medicine samples and the clinic had a sizable initial stock. This is a standard practice with private practice doctors, but the need was much more critical in a clinic that would serve many patients who could not afford most prescribed medicines. In addition, they donated office supplies and patient forms. It may seem trivial, but an item easily taken for granted such as a clipboard becomes a welcome and essential gift with a full waiting room on opening day and every patient is trying to complete several forms. Some drug companies made small cash grants that helped fill unanticipated gaps.

Within a few weeks of his return from Sri Lanka, Dr. Kim had moved from disappointed dreamer to a man frenetically executing a mission. With the help of the great staff of The Foundation, progress was underway on the building renovation and a sound financial management system was in place. Dr. Kim was concentrating on recruiting doctors, nurses, and administrative volunteers. He also was coordinating support from Lab Corp and drug company reps. There were hundreds of details that had to be addressed, but the major thread running through all this action was to do the most important things first. That is, just do what it takes to get the clinic open, the details will take care of themselves.

TAKING SOME RISKS

Letting the details take care of themselves can be a risky business. On the athletic field, risk might result in a bruised limb or ego, but the reward is often worth it. The Fosbury Flop was risky the first time it was tried in public. Yet, it completely changed high jumping and is an example of taking a risk and reaping the rewards. Athletics is one thing and medicine is entirely another. So, lest the clinic's approach be misconstrued as a lack of concern and a careless attitude toward the serious business of operating a clinic, what risk taking meant to the clinic planners will be clarified.

The approach of "just do what it takes to get the clinic open, the details will take care of themselves" makes sense when it is clear that it applies only to the administrative details of the clinic. One simple example is the numbering of patient charts. When a committee handles an issue like this, it may take some time to arrive at an agreement on the best way to do it. While there are many efficient and effective ways to complete this necessary and important task, the Free Clinic planners chose to let this detail take care of itself.

Rather than spend precious time solving a minor problem, planners tabled this issue almost until the first patient arrived. Shortly before that point, someone said let's number them sequentially and that became the method. Nothing complex, just start with number "1" and keep on going. This simple approach proved to be effective and had some unexpected benefits in the "purely paper" operation that emerged in the clinic. Want to know how many patients the clinic has treated? Look at the last file number and that will be close enough. (More rigorous methods were used for any official patient count data.) It worked out that postponing the chart numbering issue to concentrate on more critical actions was a good decision.

In many ways, the point to be made here is that the clinic planners were not arbitrary and careless in what they chose to defer. They had made rationale decisions to let some things wait. They felt very responsible for getting the major things right. They knew they could not make any fatal errors and recover. But, how to know what is a fatal error? When should planners address an issue in agonizing detail in order to get it right? The overall criterion when deciding how much detail to cover before proceeding was to error on the side of caution.

Implementing this principle of caution was a very practical exercise. What follows is a wide ranging discussion of the clinic's approach to deciding what must be done and how it must be accomplished.

First, it was very important to know the rules. One example is the Tennessee Good Samaritan Law. The State Legislature has offered some level of protection to medical personnel offering free care. (Without pretending to be a legal or definitive explanation of the statute, it basically says that any physician practicing without compensation can not be sued, except for gross negligence.) Knowing and explaining this to potential volunteer doctors greatly helped in recruiting. Many doctors did not know they had this protection. Knowing the rules in this case was essential so that this very important detail could be handled properly.

A formal learning session coordinated by The Foundation provided this important information to potential medical volunteers. On June 22, 2005, approximately six weeks before the first patient arrived at the expanded free clinic, a dinner, presentation, and Q&A session was held at the Baptist Health System facilities. More than thirty physicians were invited based upon their expressed interest in helping at the clinic and twenty were able to attend the meeting. To have not addressed this issue formally with the doctors would have been a fatal error.

In brief, the agenda included presentations by a Tennessee State Senator familiar with the law and the legislature's intent, an attorney with experience defending malpractice cases, and a senior hospital administrative executive. These three individuals were able to speak authoritatively, practically, and in depth about this subject. This meeting was instrumental in relieving a major concern of most medical professionals. As in South Carolina, a single malpractice insurer effectively covers Tennessee and general information concerning their procedures was discussed. Clinic planners made every effort to ensure they knew and shared the rules with volunteer physicians.

Knowing the basic non-profit rules was also fundamental. The Free Clinic needed and sought the special status conferred by Section 501(c) (3) of the IRS Code. While most of the planners had a general understanding of a non-profit, the distinction of a federal tax exempt organization, and the effort required to obtain it, was not clear. The planners needed to know the rules and quickly learned them with the help of The Foundation and a private attorney. The route to state tax exempt status, which effectively reduced the cost of anything the clinic purchased, is another example of the importance of knowing the rules.

The list of rules for a clinic is important long and complex. It also varies with organizational structures and within different states. The point here is not to exhaustively identify what rules a potential clinic must know, but to emphasize that when fast tracking it is extremely important to know the rules. It is impossible to take only reasonable risks without understanding the rules that define those risks. The color of the paint in the waiting room is of no real consequence. The chemical composition of that paint may be of great consequence and adequately assessed only by knowing the rules.

Second, imbedded in the clinic planners' approach was the notion that asking for advice was always important. For example, you can never know the rules if you don't ask what the rules are. As noted, there were many sources of advice. The planners sought advice and counsel from The Foundation, individual doctors and nurses, hospital administrators, attorneys, and many others. But, a part of moving forward is to ask, "How can I do this?" There is a world of difference between asking, "<u>Can</u> the clinic do this," and "<u>How</u> can the clinic do this?" Everyone learned early on that the first response often included a case for why something couldn't be done. The clinic planners were past that point.

When seeking advice, they respectfully made it clear that they had considered the situation and the reasons not to do something and the question was how to accomplish the task at hand. It was gratifying to see that most individuals and organizations responded with something along the lines of, "Since you are serious about this, here's what I would advise." The object of the exercise was to determine where fatal risks lay. The focus of the advice sought was to make a list of the things that <u>must</u> be accomplished immediately to avoid excessive risks. With this aim, the list of absolute necessities became more manageable.

The third way to avoid a fatal error was simply never to be anything less than professional. Remaining professional at all times is a difficult task. What is the difference between a passionate advocate and a rabble-rouser? How were the clinic planners to elicit the community support required without stepping on some toes? The basic message has to be that the community is not doing enough to provide for its neediest. How does one deliver this message in less than an accusatory tone?

The Free Clinic planners do not claim to have mastered this aspect of risk taking. To make no one uncomfortable and to accept every "No" is to ensure no progress. To push too hard may also end in failure. However, there were some guidelines to make things less troublesome. The planners tried to always have hard, supportable facts as to the need. This allowed them to state the need without blaming anyone. Fifty million individuals without health insurance is a powerful argument that becomes even more effective when translated to fifty-five thousand in the local community. Documenting the need avoids, to some degree, the need to explain its cause or what others have done to relieve it.

The assertion that the local medical society appears to be doing nothing is not a particularly relevant argument when approaching doctors about volunteering. To imply that doctors, as individuals or as a group, are not doing enough is not a professional approach. To state the need and present an opportunity to deal with it is much more persuasive. As an aside, the local medical association had no formal program when the Free Clinic was struggling for support, but, within a year of the clinic's opening, it had a program that cooperated extensively with the Free Clinic to provide specialty care to clinic patients. This cooperation may not have been possible if the clinic had burned too many bridges in the early days.

The clinic planners also learned that flexibility was important. Sometimes this was as simple as letting a nurse work as an administrative volunteer until comfortable with the clinic operation. Expecting a nurse to volunteer only as a nurse, even when that is the clinic's greatest need, is a lack of flexibility that limits the clinic overall. The clinic must welcome all support as offered and hope folks grow into larger roles. One retired physician has never practiced as a volunteer doctor, but has contributed significantly as an administrative volunteer. Professionalism demands flexibility.

Learning not to take things personally was also a lesson that the clinic planners had to learn. A professional does not take every objection to a proposed project as directed at them as an individual or to the value of the project. Many folks did not support the clinic for what to them were sound reasons. When carefully examined, these objections usually made sense in the particular, though not in the general. Many people are simply overextended financially, in their time commitments, and in other ways. Their refusal had nothing to do with the worth of the clinic. To allow for this view is wise. Not to allow for this possibility and to react in haste or frustration entails the risk of making unnecessary enemies.

Avoiding the risk of unprofessional behavior is a balancing act. It may mean not taking no for an answer. The clinic planners learned usually not to accept the first "no." Would they accept the second or the fifth? This is where judgment and experience are important. The balancing act is to determine when being just a little more persistent will result in a yes, and when it will result in no possibility of support and, worse, in a complete rejection of the clinic. It might be fitting to say that the planners were loath to accept no, but to do no harm to the clinic was their first concern.

Closely related to the idea of professionalism is the position taken toward apparent competition. To deny that there is competition for a limited amount of community support for non-profits is not realistic. Even the most generous donors cannot support every request they receive. They must necessarily pick and choose. This gives way to the zero sum game thinking that whatever one organization receives must come from what other organizations would have received. Thus it often follows that older organizations will view a new clinic as competition.

The Free Clinic planners tried to take the high road by stressing that they were not in competition with anyone. Their only interest was serving the uninsured. A recurrent theme became that the need was so great it was clear that more resources were necessary. There was both statistical and anecdotal proof that the demand for medical care for the uninsured far outweighed the supply. Nothing would make the Free Clinic happier than to go out of business because there was no need for their services, but it was not a hard sell to convince most folks of the current need.

Once that need was clear in the community's mind, the planners stressed the special contribution that the Free Clinic would make. The clinic by design would have a very lean operation. It would not have sophisticated diagnostic equipment and specialists. Rather it would concentrate on primary care and refer advanced care cases to others. In this sense, the clinic would operate more as a triage facility. It would be the battalion aid station on the front-line referring more serious cases to a nearby MASH. It would treat those it could and move others on to the next level.

How was this advantageous to the "competition?" For one thing, it relieved a great deal of pressure on other facilities. The thousands of patients seen by the clinic that just required a course of antibiotics to cure a relatively minor illness now did not overload other waiting rooms. Clinic patients requiring maintenance care for chronic illness such as diabetes and hypertension could also receive that regular care at the new clinic and thus free up capacity elsewhere. Even while performing a triage function, the clinic would also handle many hundreds of episodic and continuing care cases that would undoubtedly have landed on existing providers' doorsteps.

More to the point, the Free Clinic could do it cheaper. They could do it cheaper not because they were better, but because they were different. This clinic had virtually no overhead costs. It had no administrative personnel collecting small co-pays or writing grant requests and filing reports. It avoided all Billing and Insurance Related (BIR) costs. This lean operation was limiting in some ways, but it kept overall costs low. Cost per patient was low, so for every dollar spent the clinic delivered measurably more medical care to the uninsured than if it were not in the mix. The logic became that supporting the Free Clinic leveraged the total value of medical care delivered in the community. By dividing the same "supply" pie in a slightly different manner, the "delivery" pie was actually increased. The clinic argued that any contribution was an investment that benefited the entire community.

The first folks to buy into this concept were the local hospital administrators. For example, based on the location of the clinic, Baptist Health System saw that many of the clinic's most likely patients would otherwise seek treatment in their emergency room. The potential savings in costs that must be written-off were significant. The notion of leverage – tens of dollars to support the clinic could save hundreds of dollars in ER costs made sense. The point here is not an economic analysis of ER operations, but rather to point out that Baptist Health System quickly embraced the Free Clinic as a partner not a competitor.

Not everyone in the local medical community was so eager to accept the clinic as a true partner. Many did initially view the clinic as a competitor. Most changed their minds as the clinic swung into full operation and other providers were able to refer some of their unserved clients to the Free Clinic. The clinic was eventually viewed as a full partner in serving the uninsured. This transition was easier because the clinic never viewed others as competition. Instead, clinic planners concentrated on explaining how the need was so great that many different providers must do their part, many serving in "niche markets" like the Free Clinic.

Proceeding with an aggressive attitude is not a frivolous choice. Simply trusting everything will work out is not a feasible approach. Rather, the definition of fast tracking (or just doing it) is distinguishing between fatal and non-fatal errors. This means insuring patients have the best possible care while maintaining the highest legal and ethical standards. Do these things and do them well. But, don't get wrapped around the axle with minor details. Move ahead with the faith that conscientious folks can work out the myriad of "minor" details along the way. Always move forward, but error on the side of caution.

HELP ALONG THE WAY

The clinic had moved from the dream of one man to the corporate vision of a small group of clinic planners. The clinic planners realized early on that no matter how motivated they or Dr. Kim might be, they could not do it alone. They needed a great deal of help along the way. The circle of committed backers was expanding and those willing to provide substantial support increasing. As mentioned earlier, The Foundation and Baptist Health System were instrumental in bringing the clinic to fruition. One purpose of this story is to encourage others who might want to start a new community clinic and to give them a potential road map for that journey. A detailed explanation of the critical support, characterized as "help along the way," may serve that purpose.

The actual clinic facility was the dentist office next to Dr. Kim's private practice office. The go ahead on remodeling from The Foundation cleared the way to start work. A working budget of around $20,000 made plans to quickly convert the space doable. A dentist's office and a medical clinic share many features in common—reception area, a waiting room, records storage, and similar functional spaces. Other parts are not comparable. For example, a dentist will normally have treatment rooms with a dental chair and extensive water, pressurized air, and other specific requirements. A medical exam room generally requires an exam table and less specialized equipment and support. Privacy is a major concern in a medical exam room where some dentists function in open areas.

So, starting with the common features the contractor designed a clinic that capitalized on the existing configuration. The clinic had two exam rooms, a hematology station and lab to draw blood and process specimens, a records storage area/supply room that also afforded some privacy for weighing patients, a doctor's office/work space, a glass walled receptionist's cubicle with counter, and a ten patient waiting room. A contractor did the major work, but volunteers did some things to help hold down costs. For example, a volunteer built and painted the patient records shelves after the major renovation work.

The completed office space made it easier to visualize the furniture and equipment required to operate the clinic. Nothing is quite as bare or appears as large as an empty waiting room. One clinic supporter visited and saw the need for waiting room furniture. She set about solving that problem and soon the clinic had a furnished waiting room with chairs, end tables, and plants. The room did not appear as spacious as before, but it was welcoming and functional.

Exam tables and medical equipment came from Baptist Health System through the efforts of The Foundation. Most lab equipment was donated by Lab Corp as part of their support of testing services. An individual donor gave telephone equipment. Other local health care providers also helped. Fort Sanders Hospital, a unit of Covenant Health, provided office furniture and other material support. In-kind donations were frequent and helped to prepare the clinic for its planned opening.

The physical amenities and setup were well underway, but the operational procedures of the clinic were not clearly addressed at this point. Again The Foundation took the lead in shepherding the clinic through the process of establishing a concept of operations. The administrative support required by even the most basic medical clinic is enormous. At a high level, the basic requirements for any patient visit would consist of making an appointment, completing paperwork, treatment, follow-up, and record keeping. Someone must make plans to meet these requirements. The Foundation looked to their familiar hospital environment for a solution.

Planners made the decision to tie-in the clinic to the BHS IT support system by computer to provide for scheduling and basic clinic record keeping. This approach was not intended to create electronic patient health care records, but would permit collecting some basic statistical or demographic patient data such as number of visits, age, sex, etc. (The clinic would maintain all patient health records.) This meant The Foundation must arrange for voice, fax, and internet phone lines and they did. They also provided a Baptist Health System computer prior to the first administrative volunteers' arrival. Conceptually, the clinic would be prepared to make appointments through the BHS IT system on opening day.

The efforts of The Foundation staff were essential to preparing the clinic for operation and they were willing to do everything possible. They did not just drop off a computer at the clinic. They ensured it was wired in with Baptist Health System and more importantly that BHS IT personnel knew how the clinic was to operate. A partial list of the areas that The Foundation covered for the clinic includes: supplies, bookkeeping, printing, and most importantly overall advice. As noted, The Foundation had done this before.

Dena Mashburn, a Family Nurse Practitioner, serving as The Foundation's Community Health Partnership Director, had worked with a number of community clinics and similar activities and brought a wealth of experience to the clinic planners. She was able to provide a suggested list of medical supplies and went the extra mile by arranging for them to be on hand. The Foundation's administrative staff handled all purchasing, accounting, and housekeeping functions such as office supplies for the clinic. The Foundation was receiving all donations and paying the bills for the clinic at this time. If a publicity flyer or other document was needed, The Foundation arranged for the BHS Printing Office to do the work. The sheer amount of support and the level of detail furnished by The Foundation were critical to the progress the clinic made prior to opening.

The advice the clinic received from The Foundation was constant and fundamental to the success of the clinic. The Foundation staff knew the "Nike Clinic" was compelled to move forward quickly and not sweat the details. Yet, years of hospital and non-profit experience made The Foundation staff realize that many things required going by the book. For example, the requirements of the Health Insurance Portability and Accountability Act (HIPAA) are complex and demanding. Most doctors and nurses are well aware of the basic requirements, but the day to day compliance generally falls on the shoulders of administrators. As opening grew nearer, Dena looked for someone at the clinic to cover this base. She again took the responsibility and created a HIPAA form for the clinic, instructed key volunteers in its use, and ensured it was available and used.

She also suggested that some key volunteers visit other clinics in the local area prior to opening to see how they operated. These visits would qualify as benchmarking under any corporation's definition of the term. A visit to the Jefferson Rural Clinic in Jefferson City, Tennessee, proved to be the single most important event in the development of the Free Clinic's administrative operating procedures. Based on the results of an onsite visit and in-depth interviews, the need for some adjustments in the proposed concept of operations became clear. The Foundation staff concurred in these changes and once again facilitated their implementation.

Help along the way included other forms of support, some of which the clinic planners had not specifically anticipated. An answering service provides a good example of the spontaneous assistance that came forward. One lady who owned and operated a telephone answering service had read about the clinic and its mission of serving the uninsured. She was impressed with the efforts to help those in need in the community. Working at the clinic as a volunteer was not possible because her business, which was essentially a 24/7 operation, did not give her much free time. Unsolicited, she contacted Dr. Kim and told him that she was appreciative of the clinic's work and would like to help, but could not volunteer. She then offered to provide telephone answering services for the clinic free of charge.

The clinic accepted her offer and arrangements made to establish the service. Technically, the procedure of setting up an answering service was simple. A message was recorded on an assigned telephone number and clinic calls forwarded to it. While technically simple, it proved to be a critical operational step. A clinic staffed by volunteers is limited in its operational hours. Many calls will go unanswered. Forwarding calls to a recorded message, keeps the information given to the public consistent.

Clinic eligibility, operating hours, appointment procedures, and location were the first items included. As the clinic became more experienced, the message was changed several times to include important new items such as what to do if the caller is experiencing a medical emergency. A more traditional physician answering service with a "live" operator may be effective when there is an on call doctor available, but that was a luxury the clinic did not enjoy. In this case, less was more – more effective for the clinic's needs. This may seem a trivial matter, but small acts of kindness and support were essential in preparing the clinic for opening day.

The support of Baptist Health System and The Foundation included diagnostic support. Diagnostic services were critical and were in place before the first patient arrived. Baptist Health System was generous in providing these services free of charge. The Free Clinic had no diagnostic equipment, meaning that relatively simple procedures such as an X-ray or EKG would be completed at Baptist Hospital. Baptist made "Imaging Requests" and other internal forms available to the clinic and honored them without exception. For all intents and purposes, a volunteer doctor at the Free Clinic had the full range of tests available at a major hospital at his or her disposal. X-rays were available to clinic patients without an appointment. MRIs, Sonograms, and other procedures might require an appointment, but volunteers could quickly schedule them.

The close proximity of Baptist Hospital to the Free Clinic eased the diagnostic testing procedure. Many patients were able to go straight from the clinic to the hospital outpatient registration office for testing. Procedures included an agreement with a radiology group that would read the results and prepare report summaries for the Free Clinic doctors. These procedures were in place before the clinic saw its first patient and worked well with little refinement.

Knoxville is a college town with a major university. The University of Tennessee has had national collegiate championships in football and women's basketball, some as recent as 2008. To say that Knoxville is a sports town is an understatement, so it should be expected that sports metaphors often flavor the local speech. One of these is, "A good defense is the best offense," which goes back to the days of General Bob Neyland. This is also a phrase used frequently by Tom Kim when referring to his friend Wayne Kline. Wayne is a local attorney who has represented a number of physicians and Tom likes to point out that he always presents a good defense.

In addition to his courtroom skills, Wayne proved to be a special friend to the Free Clinic. He is another of the incredible folks who helped along the way. The reluctance of doctors to expose themselves to a malpractice risk is one of the major impediments to recruiting doctors for a free clinic. Wayne was there to address this issue from the first and brought a lot of peace of mind to those who saw it as a major obstacle to volunteering. The February meeting included a presentation by Wayne on the Tennessee Good Samaritan Law. His thorough presentation delivered the facts, but his stature in the community sealed the deal. Many doctors were willing to simply trust his judgment. He knew a lot about defenses and if he said "don't worry," many were willing to sign on.

In addition to removing this major hurdle to finding doctors willing to volunteer, he took on the major administrative burdens faced by the clinic at this point in its development. He knew that a charter as a 501(c) (3) was the minimum required for the clinic to move ahead. The clinic was chartered on March 3, 2005, less than a month after the February meeting at Cedar Springs Church. The IRS issued an Employer Identification Number on April 7, 2005, and confirmed the clinic's tax deductible status on March 8, 2006. Anyone familiar with non-profit organizations and IRS reporting requirements will recognize that this represents an enormous amount of work.

Wayne was a rock solid supporter of the clinic who wanted to be sure that things were done correctly. Just as Baptist Health System and The Foundation did everything possible to avoid fatal errors, he took the same responsibility upon himself. In most cases, rather than waste time explaining why something was needed, he simply took action and ensured it was correct. Wayne eventually became the Chair of the Board of Directors of the Free Clinic and continues to serve in that capacity as this story is being written. It is hard to imagine the clinic in its current form without the contributions of Wayne Kline. Working at risk is practical only when someone is minding the store and making sure the critical bases are covered.

The run-up to the clinic opening was as a balancing act between "just getting things done" and "don't make a fatal error." Concentrate on the later and the clinic will never open because there will always be another detail or problem to solve. Concentrate on the former and the clinic may open, but soon find itself in hot water. In this instance well-meaning individuals will have done more harm than good.

It appears the Free Clinic did a satisfactory job of balancing these opposing factors. In what were really only a few short weeks, the clinic planners were ready to announce opening day. D-Day was Monday, August 1, 2005. On that date the new clinic would welcome the first patient. Dr. Kim, clinic planners, and those special folks who helped along the way poured a tremendous amount of hard work into opening the clinic. They had also given a great deal of themselves. Their hopes and dreams were riding on this venture. With so much invested and so much preparation, things just had to go smoothly.

That was not exactly the case. The most that can be said is that fatal flaws were avoided. There were no disasters, but it was now time to thoroughly address the many "small" tabled items. As the volunteer pool expanded beyond the small core group that operated under the get the important things done principle, many folks began to ask questions. Some were as basic as, "What do I say when someone calls to make an appointment?" These questions required clear, specific answers. The narrative now turns to the first days of the clinic's operation and how the "minor decisions" delayed for sometime became important issues and for immediate resolution.

Five Fingers

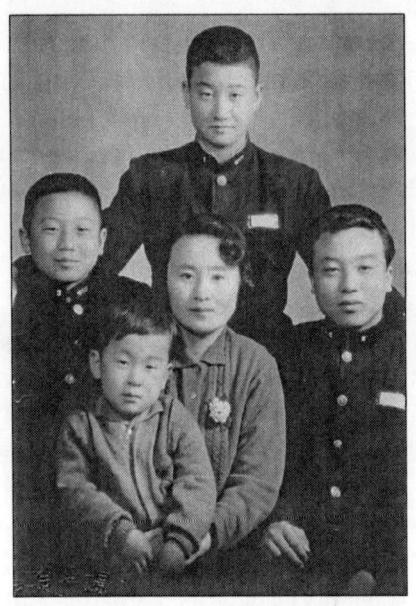

Tom Kim (top center) as a teenager in Korea.

Five Fingers

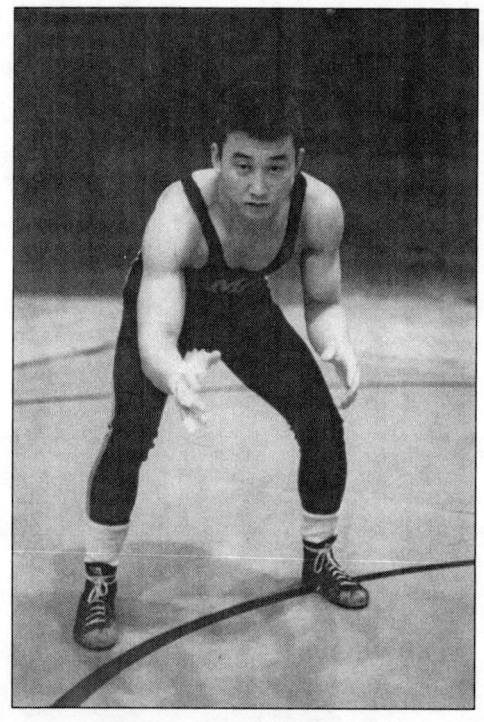

The Wrestler who wouldn't quit.

Five Fingers

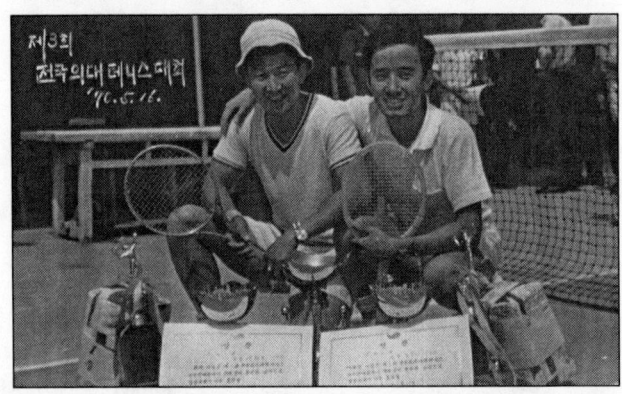

Tom Kim (left) Korea National Collegiate Tennis Champ with his doubles partner Bwung B. Park. Dr. Park is now Chair of Plastic Surgery Department, Yongsei University Medical School.

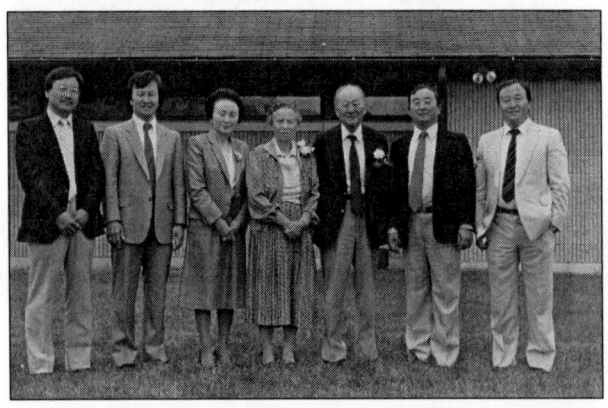

The Kim family in Dayton, Ohio during Tom's medical training in 1977.
From left to right: Harry, Tom, Hyun, Mrs. Soon Kim, Dr. Bong Oh Kim, Paul, and Sam.

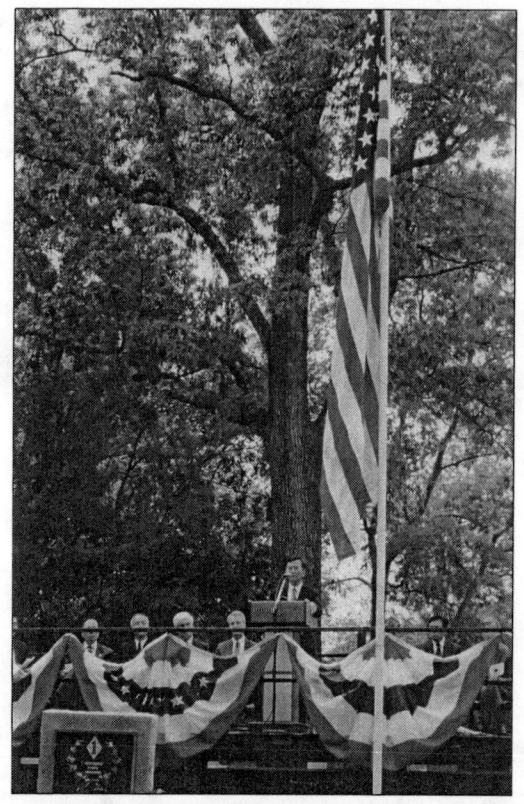

Tom Kim speaking at the dedication of the
Korean War Veteran's Monument
in Knoxville, Memorial Day, 2003

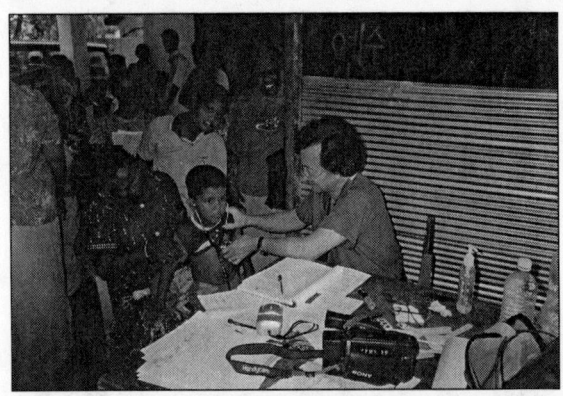

Dr. Tom Kim providing medical care as part of the Tsunami Disaster Relief in Sri Lanka, March, 2005

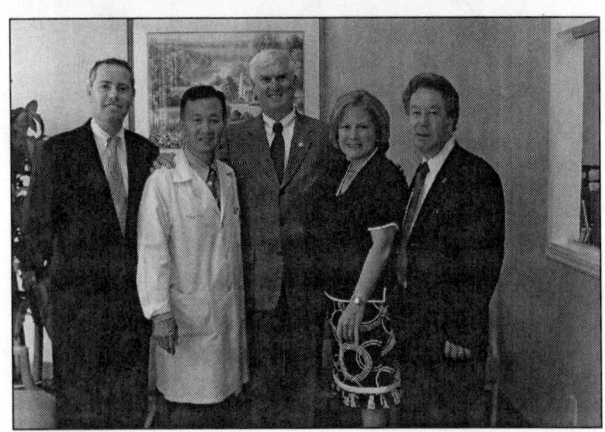

Congressman Jimmy Duncan and Terry Morgan, CEO, Baptist Health System Foundation, participate in August, 2005 opening of the Free Clinic. From left to right: Dean Rice, Tom Kim, Rep. Duncan, Ms Morgan, and Bob Griffitts

Five Fingers

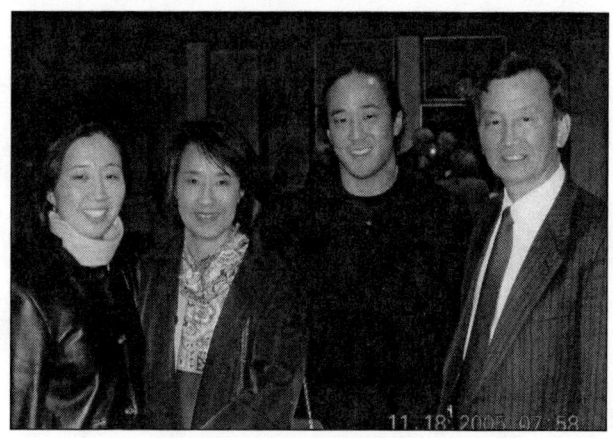

The Kims at the November 2005
Community Update.
From left to right: Kimberly, Hwa, Tim, and Tom.

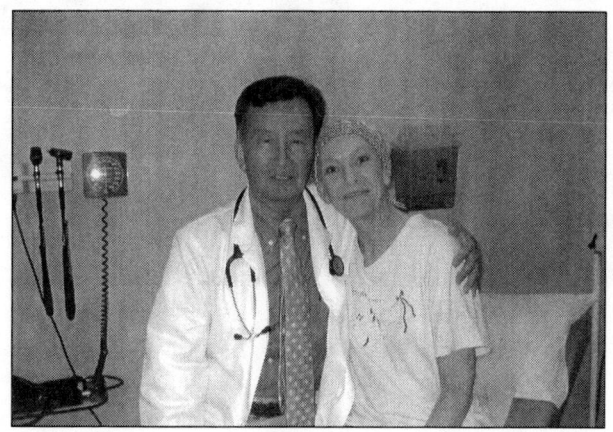

Dr. Tom Kim with a Clinic Patient

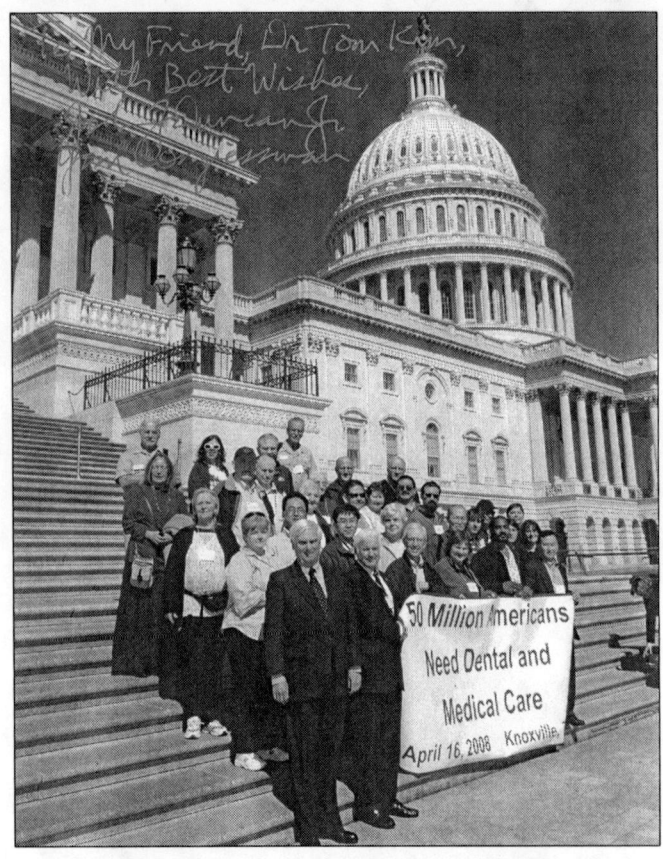

Clinic patients and supporters rally on
Capitol steps in Washington DC
to raise awareness of the uninsured in America,
April, 2008.

Five Fingers

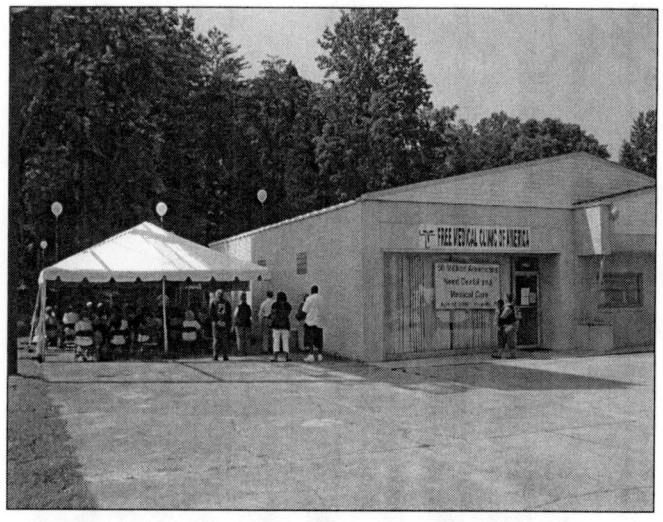

The Free Clinic celebrates its fourth anniversary and 20,000th appointment in 2009.

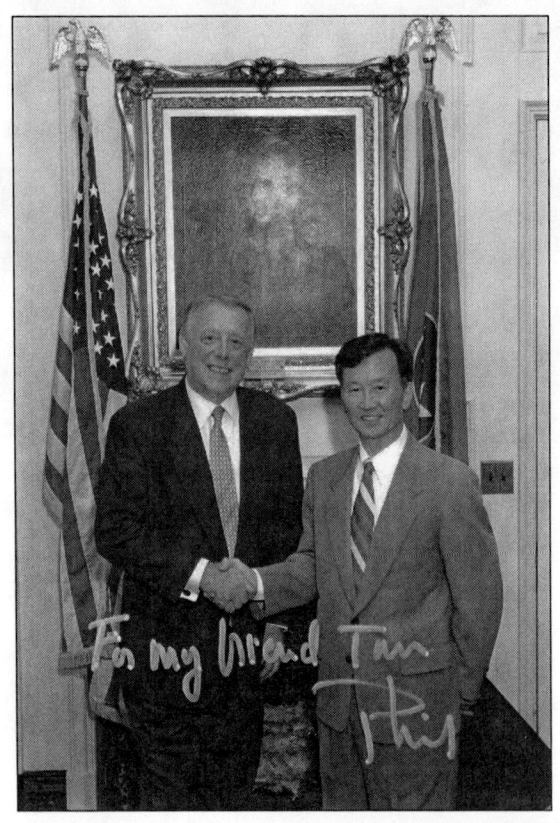

Dr. Tom Kim with Tennessee Governor Bredesen.

THE DAYS

Counting from the February meeting at Cedar Springs Church, the clinic planners had worked for less than six months toward the opening of the clinic. They accomplished a great deal in that relatively short period of time. Doctors and nurses had been recruited. A new clinic facility had been prepared. Medical supplies had been laid in. Basic office equipment – phones, a computer, file cabinets, furniture, forms, folders, etc., had been assembled. Some office and administrative volunteers had been recruited. Was the clinic ready to go?

Not by a long shot! The gist of fast tracking is to delay the less important or more mundane decisions so that the really critical ones can be attacked head-on. Now was the time to address the minor decisions. What does a patient folder look like? How will it be numbered or identified? How will patient records be filed and retrieved? The list of administrative questions that had been delayed, for very good reasons, was long and complex. There was nothing left undone that would prevent the clinic from opening because it had a solid administrative foundation. However, there was a lot to be done to put the clinic in order for the first patient.

August 1, 2005, was the first day for patients. It was fast approaching and to some degree the clinic planners were still advancing almost entirely on faith. Help had appeared when most needed on the major issues and they sensed that the same might be the case in the last weeks. This final run-up focused on administrative details and some of the problems were unknowns at this stage. The story of the first few days of the Free Clinic is the story of how some key folks found their way to the clinic and assembled the final pieces of the puzzle. There was much to be done and not a lot of time. But everything was completed and the chaotic first few days of the clinic's operation shaped and molded much of the final course of the clinic.

Frenetic activity filled the last two weeks before Opening Day. It was during this period that many operating principles were set and the character of the clinic was determined. A strict chronological account of these days does not tell the complete story because many things were being done in parallel, but it does allow for the key events to be placed chronologically and their impact explained.

On Sunday, July 3, 10, and 17, 2005 the following notice appeared in the worship announcement at Cedar Springs Presbyterian Church:

Volunteers needed for free medical clinic. Dr. Tom Kim is opening a free medical clinic at 6209 Chapman Highway this month. This clinic will provide vital health care for those who cannot afford it. Volunteer positions include doctors, nurse-practitioners, nurses, administrative workers, front-desk helpers, and cleaning crew. To volunteer or for more information, call Dr. Kim's office (577-5561).

The individuals who called were invited to sign up for a day to begin work. Details would be provided at the first session. A number of church members responded and formed the first wave of administrative volunteers.

At the same time, volunteers came from many sources other than Cedar Springs. Dr. Kim and the clinic planners had many contacts and had secured commitments from several individuals with medical administrative experience. For example, a number of hospital volunteers from Baptist Hospital had signed up and were available. Several more churches, particularly those in South Knoxville, heard of the clinic and its needs. They provided a number of volunteers, often from a single Sunday School Class or similar group.

The medical aspects of the clinic were well in hand, but the administrative details were not complete. The administrative volunteers became known as "office volunteers." Their primary duties were to verify eligibility, make appointments, serve as receptionists during clinic treatment hours, and in-process patients. Office volunteers became the face of the clinic – the first to greet patients and the last to wish them well as they left the clinic.

The appointment making process started with determining if an individual was eligible for care by the clinic. The clinic's eligibility was a carry over from the after-hours clinic. In short, a Free Clinic patient must 1) be employed, 2) have no health insurance, and 3) be a US citizen or permanent resident. These criteria had served well before and they remain in effect today. Dr. Kim felt he could treat four patients an hour. These two guidelines, eligibility and patient load, formed the core of the procedural guidance that would be available to the first office volunteers. It was time for a special person to appear and she did.

Laura Lee Needham had responded and volunteered for the first day of scheduling patients. She showed up at the clinic and was briefed by Janis Sims, Dr. Kim's Assistant Office Manager. (Janis would be next door helping to run Dr. Kim's private practice until September 2006 and was an invaluable resource for the clinic during its entire first year.) Laura Lee took the two available administrative guidelines and sprang into action. She decided to record appointments in a "Week At-a-Glance" appointment book. This format broke the days of the week into 15 minute blocks by hour and was a logical way to meet the patient load criteria. The eligibility requirements were explained over the phone to each prospective patient. With little more than this, Laura Lee answered the major "how" questions and, in effect, established the basic administrative procedures for the clinic. No committees, no best practices, no consultants. There was a task at hand and Laura Lee was a get it done type person.

That first day answered many questions. A few phone calls taught Laura Lee that potential patients still had many unanswered questions. She quickly developed standard answers. Patients must have positive identification, so bring a photo Id and a driver's license certainly fit that bill. Patients must prove their employment, so bring a pay stub or similar proof. If you are on medication, bring a list. The clinic did not need extensive information to make an appointment, but name and phone number were the minimum. Be sure and give directions to the clinic. Laura Lee had created a rudimentary telephone script for the clinic, although it was not yet reduced to writing.

In addition to establishing the basic appointment making procedures for the clinic, Laura Lee adopted the clinic as her personal mission. She assumed responsibilities far beyond those expected from an office volunteer. She became the "go to person" for the clinic. She devoted an enormous amount of time working out operational details and working on-site with volunteers assisting them during the first weeks of operation. She was the first volunteer with a clinic key because she often opened and closed the clinic. In the earliest days of the clinic, the most common answer to an office volunteer's question was, "Ask Laura Lee." The second most frequent was, "Ask Janis." Dr. Kim was fully engaged with the medical aspects of the clinic; and, by in large, administrative details were left to Laura Lee.

The second day of clinic operations continued the pattern of the first. No patients had been treated, but the clinic was experiencing solid demand for appointments. The time slots in the clinic calendar were filling up. To some degree the need for the clinic had been assumed and that assumption was quickly validated. Now, the next group of volunteers showed up and were briefed. This briefing was easier because there was a pattern to follow. The calendar was there to show how to schedule an appointment. The first day's experience had refined the telephone script. Janis used the tried and true method of "watch me do the first one" to teach the lessons learned.

The phone was removed from call forwarding and the clinic was again in live operation. Janis answered the first call, effectively and efficiently covering the required points, and entered a new appointment. She stayed around for the second call and when convinced the new volunteers had mastered the procedure, left for her office with the assurance she would quickly return if needed. The second day was underway without any major mishaps and the calendar serving as an appointment book was showing signs of heavy use.

A look around the clinic office showed many things were missing. There was a computer, but no printer. There were phone lines, but no fax. There was an apparent need to copy patient documents, but no copier. It was obvious there were still equipment needs.

The search was on for this basic office equipment. The option of purchasing a "three-in-one" printer, fax, and copier was an easy choice. One was located that seemed to meet the clinic's needs. It then became clear that the clinic had no purchasing procedures for an item that cost more than a few dollars or was not in the BHS supply system. No one knew how to buy a major item. It took considerable effort to actually make the purchase, but it did point the way to a more efficient method. The clinic refined the process over the next few weeks. The small, fragile HP machine, designed for home, not commercial use, did not appear to be up to the demands of a bustling clinic. A note saying "treat me gentle, no large copying jobs" was placed near the feeder tray in hopes of limiting its use. Almost four years later, that same machine serves the clinic with only one short pause for repair.

With the arrival of the three-in-one printer, work on setting up the office could proceed. As mentioned, the only IT equipment on hand was a desk top computer and monitor. The plan was that the computer would be remoted into the BHS IT network and used as a sophisticated work station able to schedule appointments, exchange documents, and generally function as if the Free Clinic were an in-house Baptist Health System operation.

The necessary voice and Fax phone lines were available, as well as an Internet connection and ISP, but nothing was connected. A clinic volunteer picked up the three-in-one device at the store and by using old cables from home was able to successfully connect it.

By trial and error, the Fax, Internet, and Printer ports were matched with the correct plugs and the clinic was ready to function. It could now send and receive a Fax, send and receive e-mail, copy documents, and print hard copy computer pages as needed. Again, there was solid ground work, but it took volunteers with a "whatever it takes attitude" to close the loop.

By the end of the week, the clinic was almost ready to function in the twenty-first century telecommunications world. The phone rang constantly, questions were answered and appointments were scheduled. Fax and computer requirements were still at a minimum, so there was no real test of those systems, but they were available. To make an appointment the only administrative action required was to write the patient's name and phone number in the appointment book. This was a relatively simple task that every volunteer could handle. There were many willing hands and several days of appointments were already booked. It appeared that things might be under control.

However, the clinic had not seen patient number one. Making an appointment is the easy part of the administrative process. Receiving, in-processing, treating, and closing the visit are the really difficult parts. Because the first two weeks did not involve interacting with patients, the clinic planners and volunteers simply did not know what they did not know. Planners made grand plans of how the single computer would automate patient related tasks, but just did not understand the problems involved. So, except for resolving a few minor issues such

Five Fingers

as making copies, a workable in-processing procedure did not exist. Once patients arrived, the need for specific, consistent, standard procedures would become clear.

The details of the process improvements are covered in the next chapter. It was only after the first few weeks of patient appointments that the range and depth of the adjustments required were clear. In one sense the administrative preparation for the first patients was complete by the third day. The appointment procedures that were set and refined on the first two days became the standard operating procedure for the clinic.

However, there was much more than making appointments to concern Dr. Kim. He began to rely on a small group of office volunteers as he identified problems and sought solutions. He would ask certain volunteers to "take care of ..." and they would respond. To promote consistency in clinic operations many procedures were rapidly reduced to writing. As the clinic developed its first set of basic operating procedures, office volunteers were expected to follow this more specific written guidance. For some this was a learning experience. For others, it required skills they did not have or had not yet perfected. As a result, there was a lot of variation in how office volunteers performed their basic duties.

Again, a small group of volunteers agreed to lead an effort to have an experienced, knowledgeable individual at the clinic as much as possible. They divided the days of the week among themselves with each taking responsibility for a day or two of the week to ensure someone was there to provide structure and explain new procedures to office volunteers. They also met regularly to discuss the challenges they saw and propose solutions. They were, in effect, a steering committee for clinic administrative operations. The clinic had no full or part-time employees for almost its first two full years. Volunteers assumed all the duties of an office manager.

As a survival technique, the unofficial steering committee, headed by Laura Lee, adopted a division of labor plan. Laura Lee assumed the duties of unofficial office manager, doing whatever it took to keep things running, including handling a plumbing emergency. Another volunteer became responsible for scheduling and coordinating nurses and office workers. Two retirees agreed to try to develop some administrative procedures, the supporting documentation, and handle any reporting requirements. These willing volunteers enjoyed their work, but also learned that when an aggressive approach is embraced things will move fast and folks must be willing to step up and fill needs as they arise.

Without an office manager who could be on-site day in and day out, this system just emerged as an expedient to meet the needs at hand. The decision to do things quickly and open the clinic without any paid administrative staff generated the need for volunteers willing and able to go beyond the basics. Many folks accepted the challenge, and no one was happier when an office manager was hired than the members of the "unofficial steering committee."

During the final preparation before seeing patients, office volunteers made only administrative contributions. They were not qualified or willing to address the medical side of operations. Planners must leave every aspect of the medical practice to the medical staff. This separation of functions is critical. Good medicine must always be the primary concern and should drive administration. The purpose of any clinic procedure must be to aid the effective delivery of medical care and never serve only bureaucratic or administrative ends.

OPENING DAY

Two weeks of making appointments passed quickly. A full schedule awaited the volunteer doctors and nurses on opening day. Excited clinic volunteers felt ready to welcome patient number one to the clinic. However, in many ways the past several days had been the calm before the storm. Laura Lee was functioning as the clinic office manager, overseeing, encouraging, and training office volunteers. She was also dealing with a myriad of details such as assembling forms, supplies, and other essentials for opening day. Again, because no patients had yet been treated, the clinic volunteers simply did not know what they didn't know.

One funny example was the assembling of a patient file or folder. The clinic planners settled on a strictly numerical folder numbering system and Dr. Kim had designated four forms for each patient file. Volunteers stapled three "permanent" forms on the left side of the folder and the remaining form was loose on the right side. There was clear method to this madness. The doctor's progress notes were frequently used, faxed and copied. Stapling the other forms prevented their loss and brought some order to the file.

The humor lies in the fact that the forms be stapled in a particular way. The staples were to head into the folder, which was exactly opposite the natural way a volunteer would handle and staple the folder. The procedure was a commonsense solution to the problem of folders hanging on one another when pulled off the shelf. A great reason for the procedure, but the rationale was unknown to the office volunteers.

During opening day and most of the first week or so, office volunteers became accustomed to Dr. Kim reminding workers of the correct stapling method. Occasionally, he would come into the receptionist cubicle and demonstrate the proper method. In any event, the staple lecture soon became a minor rite of passage for office volunteers. You were not a qualified veteran until you knew how to staple a folder. Months later, old clinic hands would still admonish new volunteers to be sure they stapled correctly.

Who would have anticipated that stapling forms in a folder was such a big deal? The point is obviously that the devil lies in the details. Many of those details remained unknown until patients arrived and were processed into the clinic. Most issues were worked out on an *ad hoc* basis. For example, now that patients and patient files were part of the daily activities, how would a volunteer find a patient file number? The immediate answer was simple and that was to record the patient name, file number, and phone number in a circular Rolodex file. At the end of opening day, each new patient would have a card alphabetically filed in the Rolodex. Volunteers completed cards for each patient every day the clinic saw patients.

This simple procedure highlights the scope of not knowing the administrative challenges to be encountered until the clinic had actual experience with patients. First, the Rolodex flew in the face of the computer standing idly by. No thought was given to an electronic solution to this problem, even though the concept of operations was still to tie the clinic into BHS IT System. In that system, a computer stored and retrieved all patient information. The assumption was this procedure would extend to the clinic theoretically simply, but practically a major task. The first indication that a remote link to BHS IT resources may not be the best solution came on opening day when the Rolodex took preference over the computer. The volunteers were learning their best laid plans might not work when put to a real life test.

Second, the impact of patient volume and throughput was unknown for some time. (Volume is how many patients and throughput is how fast they come.) A Rolodex is an elegant solution to many problems even in this hypo-technical world of blackberries and I-phones. A Rolodex with up to a few hundred patients is manageable. What do you do when it is a few thousand? Get another Rolodex. That was the experience of the clinic over time. The number of Rolodexes taking up valuable counter space increased rapidly. Each time, the solution became a newer and bigger Rolodex. It was impossible to anticipate and precisely understand this problem until the clinic began seeing patients, assigning file numbers, and storing and retrieving files by the thousands. A clinic can not know the full impact of patient volume and throughput until dealing with it on a daily basis. Once a clinic has substantial experience, it will begin to understand what could not be known on opening day.

Third, when treating thousands of patients and maintaining their records, it is important that clear and precise instructions be given and followed. A small operation can tolerate a little variation. In a large operation, variation can wreak havoc. There were precise written instructions for completing Rolodex cards, yet some office volunteers did not complete them. Those that were completed did not always have consistent information or format. Completing a card for each new patient had not yet become an ingrained part of the office volunteer routine. Recovering from no card in the Rolodex is relatively simple with tens of patients. With hundreds of patients it is much more difficult. Planners did not fully understand the impact of overlooking seemingly small steps until dealing with larger numbers of patients.

Monday, August 1, 2005, was opening day. Patient number one of the new Free Clinic was seen at 5:00 P.M. The clinic had decided upon three appointment sessions each day the clinic was open. The schedule included a morning session, from 9:00 A.M. to 12:00 Noon; an afternoon session from 2:00

to 5:00 P.M.; and an evening session from 5:00 to 7:00 P.M. Appointments were scheduled for each of these sessions as volunteer doctors were available. In the first week, eight sessions were open for patients, totaling twenty-one hours of professional medical care. There was at least one session Monday through Saturday that first week. In spite of the small problems described above, opening day and the first week was a rousing success.

Dr. Kim covered the first session, walking over from his private practice and seeing patients much as he had done in his after-hours free clinic. However, he saw these patients in a new facility with a large volunteer support staff available and several other physicians sharing the patient load throughout the week. The first two patients, folders #1 and #2, were a husband and wife. The wife had "brought" her husband. This was typical of the Free Clinic. Female patients would always outnumber male patients, and many males would be brought to the clinic by concerned spouses or female friends.

Twelve patients were treated that first evening on August 1st. Of the twelve opening day patients, six (50%) returned for a second or more visits at some time. One reporting criterion used by the clinic, is the number of patients who have two or more visits. This is important because it defines the clinic as a medical home. Half of the first session patients made the free clinic their medical home.

The second session had twenty-four patients with eleven returning for a second or more visits. The medical home rate for this session was forty-six percent, slightly lower than the first session. Clinic statistics will be covered in depth later, but these first two sessions seemed to be typical for the life of the clinic. After three and a half years of operation, the Free Clinic has a return rate of about forty-five percent and the average number of follow-up visits for returning patients is 3.3. Opening day was not only successful, but fairly well predictive of what the clinic would encounter in the days, weeks, and years ahead.

Other trends surfaced in the first ten sessions that the clinic would have to address. The Free Clinic would have to contend with a significant appointment no-show rate. Opening day had only two no-shows for their appointments (15%), but the second session on Tuesday had a no-show rate of twenty-eight percent. The number of no shows, and the rate, continued to increase. For the life of the clinic, the no show rate is around thirty percent. The no-show rate appeared to depend on several factors that might include time, day of the week, weather, and any number of other unknown reasons. This made the rate unpredictable and complicated booking patients. With a known no-show rate, over booking is one solution. Book ten and expect seven makes sense when the rate is steady. Accepting walk-ins is another coping strategy, but usually results in a patient waiting a long time to see if an opening occurs. The unpredictability of patients making their appointments complicated clinic operations and is an example of the unknowns discovered once the clinic began seeing patients.

Documentation was another lesson learned from opening day forward. The office script included telling patients to bring a photo Id and proof of employment. From the first session, a few patients would appear without the necessary documentation. Some would claim they had never been told to bring it and some would admit to forgetting. Others would produce such a wide variety of papers that it was clear they had no understanding of what they were attempting to verify. Many patients offered social security cards as "photo Ids" even though they have no photograph. The most difficult task was to try to determine if the problem was one of misunderstanding or an attempt to beat the system.

By far, most patients cheerfully, and in some cases proudly, produced a driver's license and paycheck stub. The few who could not caused an excessive workload and a certain amount of confusion among office volunteers. As explained with Rolodex cards, it is important that clear and precise instructions be given and followed. Frankly, many office volunteers substituted their own interpretation of the eligibility criteria and tried to enforce it. This made for an inconsistent application of the rules to say the least. However, documentation of eligibility, which was assumed to be a straight forward task, proved to be very difficult when dealing directly with patients. It certainly was another unknown revealed on opening day.

Opening day also taught some positive lessons. Chief among them was the gratitude of most patients for the service provided. Almost without exception, patients were profusely and sincerely appreciative of the clinic and its service. Some tears were shed that first day because twelve individuals felt somebody cared and they knew they had found a medical home they could count on. Though advertised and promoted as a "free" clinic, many patients asked how much they owed, expecting a co-pay or a sliding scale fee. When told they owed nothing, their smiles increased and some asked about making a contribution. The stereotype of an ungrateful, self-entitled individual was not to be found at the Free Clinic on opening day.

The second positive lesson was that the clinic planners had guessed correctly about the need. By opening day, appointments were booked several days in advance. However, the comments of the twelve patients treated the first day confirmed to some degree a Free Clinic patient profile. They told essentially the same story. They worked, couldn't afford health insurance, and didn't qualify for any assistance. Generally speaking, in America, health care is not a serious problem for the very rich or the very poor. Those in the middle do have a problem and the lower strata of that group have the most severe needs. Some working poor must daily choose between food and health care.

The stories told by opening day patients verified that many people simply don't know how they will handle a sickness or injury. Some do turn to emergency rooms. Some simply do nothing. Several patients said, "I just don't know what I would do without something like this clinic." While statisticians may classify the data as merely anecdotal, the desperation and hopelessness in some patient's voices clearly validated the need for another free community clinic. Any one in the clinic that first day, or on any subsequent day, knew there was a local need for access to health care and that this need was clear beyond a shadow of a doubt.

A final positive lesson from opening day was that volunteers found the work meaningful. They could tell from the beginning that a need was there and they were helping meet it. The kinks were not out of the system yet, but the positives far outweighed the negatives. The grateful faces that left the clinic proved the value of the service delivered. The volunteers, particularly the office volunteers experiencing their first day of clinical service, were happy and looking forward to the prospect of their next opportunity. Not a single volunteer quit during that first week. On the contrary, many now had a positive story to tell and the number of volunteers increased.

Opening day and the first week was behind Dr. Kim, and the clinic planners. "Live" operations with real patients had revealed many unanticipated nuances to operations of the expanded free clinic. Now the team began to identify needed process improvements. They rapidly made those improvements as the days turned into weeks. There were some major course corrections along with minor tweaking of operations; but, with a solid foundation in place, all the necessary elements of a sustainable venture were in place.

THE WEEKS

The clinic was off and running having completed its first week of ten sessions. The clinic saw a total of ninety-three patients that first week, including two with follow-up visits for a total of ninety-five medical encounters. During the second week, and for several weeks to follow, the emphasis turned to improving the clinic operations, making it more efficient, and dealing with the unanticipated requirements. During this "shakedown cruise," trial and error often proved to be the best way to find an answer to the many questions raised by volunteers.

First remote IT operations were not working out. The operational IT principle had been to link the Free Clinic to BHS IT and use their resources. The link was delayed for sound reasons and temporary measures, like the Rolodex, implemented. As it became clearer that a decision was necessary, the clinic sought the counsel of The Foundation. Having already coordinated the hardware and connectivity with the BHS IT system, their only additional suggestion was to benchmark operations with an area clinic they knew had an exceptional web-based computer operation.

As a result, two clinic office volunteers made the ninety minute trip up Interstate 40 to Jefferson City, Tennessee to visit the Jefferson Rural Clinic (JRC). Their primary mission was to study the clinic's administrative procedures, concentrating on computer operations and integration. In a word, the volunteers' reaction was "Wow!" This clinic had done IT right. To make a long story manageable, a retired computer entrepreneur had relocated to the Jefferson City area and through the United Way became a founding member of the JRC board. He set up a web-based system that allowed completion of appointments, volunteer schedules, and a host of other functions online from any internet connected computer. For example, a patient could log on and see available appointment date and times. Volunteers could see who was working and schedule their own work hours.

Computers were used in virtually all administrative tasks, to include transcribing doctor's notes. All this was relatively user friendly and, to prevent accidental corruption of files, the data stored behind a firewall. More important than setting up the system, the computer guru was available 24/7 to remotely maintain the system from home. All volunteers had required training before working at the clinic and did not have full access to the system until they demonstrated mastery of the basics. After spending several hours with the Free Clinic volunteers the gentleman offered to create a similar system for the Free Clinic. He would do it for free if server space and mainte-

Five Fingers

nance were available, but not for several months due to his busy schedule.

The Free Clinic volunteers returned home duly impressed and hopeful of using a similar system. Again, to make a long story short, the Free Clinic rejected the notion of a system like JRC or any highly computerized system of any sort. A decision was made to be basically a paper operation. As strange as it may sound, this was indeed the best decision for the clinic at the time. The reasoning that supported this decision was fourfold. First, the clinic couldn't wait. The clinic had almost one hundred patients in just the first week and a consistent method to handle this workload could not wait any longer, certainly not until the first of 2006 when JRC could help.

Second, Baptist Health System, which had given so much, could not support it. Consultation with the BHS IT office, determined the server space and maintenance were just not available. They had their hands full hosting and maintaining their current programs and could not sign on to manage what to them was an unknown application. The clinic was welcome to be a remote BHS IT facility, but that was the only supportable option at that time.

Third, the clinic space and budget could not support a fully computerized system. This would require more than the single desk top machine on hand. Peripherals and accessories, such as cables, printers, etc., would mean additional unbudgeted expense. And, space was at a premium in the clinic. The small counter in the receptionist cubicle could not handle an additional piece of hardware. No other unused desk space was available. If the financial, logistic, timing, and coordination obstacles were overcome, there was simply no place to put the equipment that must be constantly in use to support appointment making, patient registration, records management, and all the other possible computerized functions. Office volunteers often asked to get rid of the one desk top computer because it took up an inordinate amount of space and seemed to serve no practical function.

The fourth, and overriding, consideration was the office volunteers themselves. The initial group of office volunteers was predominately retired folk. When asked if they could use a computer, about one half replied they didn't even know how to turn one on. As a self-characterized demographic group, the office volunteers were marginally computer literate. They were well-intended, intelligent, and active individuals who unquestionably could have learned to use a computer given the time and training. However, the clinic had started without a system in place and offered no training. If a working, user friendly system had been in place from the beginning and training available, many office volunteers would have picked it up with no problem.

The reality was that no such system was in place and it would take weeks or more to install one. The train had left the station and it was too much to ask the office volunteers to catch up. Expecting a hundred or so patient encounters a week, it seemed too great a chore to proceed in parallel – operating a paper system while simultaneously developing

Five Fingers

and installing a computer system. The impact on the office volunteer staff made the decision to go with a paper approach obvious. For what seemed excellent reasons at the time, the Free Clinic would be an old fashion paper operation.

Once the overall decision was made to go with what was on hand, the series of ensuing actions were relatively simple. The clinic completely dropped the idea of linking to BHS IT. It took steps to turn the single clinic computer into a stand alone system. This meant that some software had to be added and some minor systemic changes implemented. Baptist Health System was extremely helpful and over the years continued to help with advice, software, and site visits when necessary. (Almost four years later, the computer still thinks it is part of the BHS IT system, occasionally flashing a message to contact BHS IT office.) The computer had important uses, but they were all very simple "home-brewed" solutions.

The first, such solution was a patient roster file archiving name, address, phone number, and date of birth (DOB). Since it was for clinic use only, social security numbers were not recorded which reduced privacy concerns without limiting its effectiveness. (A link to BHS IT would require the SSN.) The EXCEL program was chosen because it could quickly calculate age using DOB and be a rudimentary database. The "Sort" function allowed compiling basic patient demographic data. Among the elements initially calculated were average and median age, gender breakdown, county of residence, and a few similar items. This information immediately proved to be very helpful in reporting to interested parties, especially current and potential donors.

The first version of the clinic roster included appointment information. After entering the first few hundred patients, it was clear the file was too large for efficient management. This led to a separate appointment file, again using EXCEL. This file proved to be extremely important because it was the source of much of the required reporting to government funding agencies, which eventually included the State of Tennessee and Knox County. It provided all the information on number of patients treated and various breakdowns of the totals. Since separated from the patient roster data, there was plenty of room to add worksheets that could respond to various requests for patient load and capacity information. Some very basic self-checking features were added to bolster confidence in the data.

Because a clinic volunteer set up the files and understood the data elements, it was easier to manipulate the data in many different ways and, to date; the system has been able to meet all information requests. Between the Roster files and the Appointment files, a volunteer could usually find a way to cross reference and compute all statistics requested. The system was not elegant, but with patience, it could be effective. It was also highly adaptive, such as when by adding a column and entering simple codes, the Roster file tracked and amassed patient TennCare data. TennCare is Tennessee's Medicaid program. Due to eligibility changes in 2005, there was great interest in identifying Free Clinic patients who previously were covered by TennCare.

The JRC visit had shown what an automated system could do. While the Free Clinic simply did not have the talent or means to duplicate it, it did learn valuable lessons and adapted them where possible. One of these lessons was the outstanding results data collected by the JRC. Each patient visit included entering a great deal of diagnostic, treatment, and disposition information. JRC shared a list of the data elements recorded and the Free Clinic developed its own limited Results file with EXCEL. The difference between JRC and the Free Clinic becomes clearer in an examination of managing results data. JRC entered it directly into a data base during the appointment. Free Clinic collected the information on a paper form and then later entered it into an EXCEL file days later. Again, it was not an elegant solution, but one that worked.

The three EXCEL files – Patient Roster, Cumulative Appointments, and Results are still used by the Free Clinic for all reporting and so far have served the clinic well. The Free Clinic method is not an optimum one. A server based, relational database is much quicker, easier, and safer. The Free Clinic simply did not have that option with its untrained volunteer base and its limited in-house computer expertise. The limited computer support of the clinic and how work-arounds were developed is not explained to endorse it as an answer for other clinics. Rather it illustrates how the trial and error process improvement method worked for this particular clinic with its unique needs and resources.

Admitting that operations would be paper based simplified process improvement in all areas. How to record appointments was one of the first tasks addressed. This process had begun with a simple weekly calendar. It was obviously not satisfactory, with the major compliant being that volunteers wrote names and numbers in very small spaces and often couldn't read their own entries. Replacing the calendar was the only option, and the sooner, the better. The steering group developed and tested several versions of an appointment calendar before accepting a final version

Office volunteers evaluated each revision and the steering committee adapted input as necessary based on feedback. The larger fonts and space for recording patient information were greatly appreciated. They made the size (legal paper) and layout (landscape) easy to settle on. The real trial and error lay in the details. Required information included name and phone number. With volunteer doctors, cancellation of an entire session's appointments, while rare, is not an unexpected event. A means of informing the patient is necessary. Some office volunteers did not recognize this necessity, and in the early days as many as one in three booked patients had no phone number recorded. For follow-up patients, file number is also helpful, but must be looked up and entered by the volunteer making the appointment. After review and testing, the final version of required information was set.

The next major adjustment was a "form follows function" argument. Appointment times could be blank and written-in by the volunteers or pre-printed as they were in the original calendar. Overbooking, no shows, and specific patient loads for specific doctors complicated this process. For example, one volunteer doctor agreed to serve at the clinic as long as he saw no more than eight patients at a session. How to ensure this request was honored, and similar requirements, was a major concern. In short what went in the time column (form) proved to have great impact on scheduling (function).

After several iterations, the compromise of having both pre-printed times and blank times was standardized. A great deal of time was spent writing and posting notes in the appointment book and overseeing scheduling in order to eliminate problems before they crept into the system. This was not always successful, with the best example being a doctor who never returned to the clinic after being overbooked with patients by well-intend, but uninformed volunteers. The final form of the appointment book was reached after several weeks of trial and error, but still requires close communication between office volunteers and clinic staff.

Of equal importance to the patient appointment book was the volunteer schedule calendar. The original all purpose calendar included office volunteers' work schedules, a procedure doomed to failure from the start. The need for a separate document was evident. It also had to meet certain other requirements: allowing volunteers to schedule themselves, clearly assigning individuals to specific functions, and indicating the doctor working that session. The first attempt was to adapt a large desktop calendar.

This did not work well so a "Staffing Calendar" was designed from scratch. It included a page for each month like a desktop calendar, but had each day of the month broken down by clinic sessions. Each session included space for specific assignments. These included the doctor assigned to duty, the assisting nurse, and the two office volunteers providing administrative support. Sessions without patients, where the only function was making appointments, required only one office volunteer and no doctor or nurse. Though cobbled together from PowerPoint slides and reproduced at a Kinkos, it was a bounded document that covered a full year and well accepted.

It was always available on the counter of the receptionist's cubicle. This allowed volunteers to sign up in advance and quickly identified uncovered sessions. Color coding doctor and nurse requirements was added. This readily identified patient treatment sessions and helped ensure a full staff was available for these sessions. The staffing calendar was developed to fill a specific need and served its purpose well. The fact that volunteers could sign themselves up had at least two concomitant benefits. It greatly reduced the number of calls the clinic volunteer coordinator had to make to ensure meeting all requirements. It also contributed directly to team building and camaraderie among the volunteers.

Office volunteers quickly settled into a routine that often included a favorite session and favorite coworker. Tuesday afternoon became "Jane's Day" and she shared it with "Susan." This gave a lot of predictability and consistency to clinic operations. These impromptu teams often quickly bonded and had significant benefits. One could flip through the staffing calendar and find the regulars signed up weeks and even months in advance. Again, a staffing calendar is not rocket science, but the steering group developed it with volunteer input and through trial and error found a format that met its needs.

Patient sign-in slips were another process that underwent improvement. Sign-in slips probably were introduced simply because they had been used in Dr. Kim's private practice. In any event, the Free Clinic began using those slips on opening day. Not designed to serve a specific purpose for the Free Clinic, they were of limited value. However, their potential as a means of keeping track of patients and capturing basic data for the Patient Roster file was recognized. The first step in process improvement was to redesign the sign-in slip to meet clinic needs. The primary purpose of the sign-in slip was to support data entry into the Roster file. The first revision rearranged data elements to facilitate data entry.

The second and third rounds added data elements such as county and TennCare status that met additional reporting needs. Also added was an employment certification, signed by the patient that affirmed their working status and that they had no health insurance. This certification, approved by an attorney, was probably of no legal consequence, but served as a good faith effort by the clinic to verify the lack of health insurance. It also had a positive reception with patients who reacted favorably when told, "We accept your word that you are not insured."

As an aside, there was no way for the Free Clinic to conveniently check that a patient had no health insurance. Local governments and hospitals could verify Medicare and TennCare status by computer; but, even for them, private insurance is a different case. Health care systems verify coverage, not the lack of it. Avoiding co-pays and deductibles are possible reasons an insured person would claim no coverage. It is probable the Free Clinic treated some insured individuals. In two or three rare cases, patients balked at signing the certification and admitted they had insurance. This probably says more about the reality that for many individuals being underinsured may be effectively the same as uninsured than about the intentions of the potential client.

The final adjustment for sign-in slips was to change the format for New and Returning patients. Some data elements were different. Different formats saved returning patients from entering data that had not changed while affording the opportunity to update any information that mattered. New and returning patient sign-in slips each had different data collection purposes and the office staff were asked to separate them. This request met with mixed results. At the next printing new slips were on yellow paper to make them more recognizable. Until the color change, some office volunteers had not known there was a difference. This was the final step in the incremental improvement process of sign-in slips.

Five Fingers

The Free Clinic had primary care as its mission. It was organized and equipped to deliver only this service. However, many patients needed more attention. The clinic certainly anticipated this requirement. Of the original fifty-seven physicians listed on the clinic's brochure as "committed to serve," thirty-two were specialists. This provided a specialty care referral resource for the clinic, but the clinic did not have standard procedures for referrals. When treating a patient at the clinic, the attending physicians could recommend referral and include this in their progress notes. The next steps were not clear, especially to the office volunteers who had an administrative role in the process.

Referrals became another process that was developed and refined early in the clinic's operation. The clinic had no full-time staff. This made tracking and monitoring referrals more difficult. The handoff of any responsibility is always a weak point in any process. When passing a file and its oversight from one worker to another, the potential for error increases dramatically. These handoffs were built into the Free Clinic's operations, with as many as three handoffs in a single day. This pointed toward a solution.

A Licensed Practical Nurse (LPN) who was volunteering as a clinical nurse saw the need and was willing to assume the responsibility for making specialty referrals. This brought structure to the process. When a doctor recommended specialty care, the patient's file was flagged and handled as a referral. The office volunteers were now responsible for two finite tasks. They must ensure a properly flagged referral file and placement in the referral inbox. The LPN would spend at least two afternoons a week processing the referrals.

As always, the medical and administrative portions of the process were separated. Only doctors made the decisions that directly impacted patient care. Dr. Kim, as clinic medical director, reviewed every referral, which required his concurrence. When required, any consultation between Dr. Kim and the referring doctor took place behind the scenes. The administrative staff only knew which referrals had been approved. Once approved, the referral process began in earnest. In short, it consisted of three steps: 1) find a specialist willing to see the patient for free, 2) make an appointment, 3) notify the patient and do everything possible to see the appointment was kept.

While the steps outlined above appear simple and straightforward they were anything but that in practice. Finding a specialist who would take a free patient soon became an issue. It was not because the specialists were unconcerned or stingy, it was because, as in most free care circumstances, demand far outstripped supply. Many specialists had committed to serve with the proviso they would limit referrals to a specific number, e.g., one per month. The stack of referrals at the Free Clinic grew rapidly and overtook the capacity of volunteer specialists in short order.

The lone LPN spent an inordinate amount of time pleading with and cajoling specialists to accept "just one more." In many cases, Dr. Kim would become involved, spending his time and goodwill, to persuade a colleague to help. The specialists contacted went well beyond the list of those who had stated their willingness to aid the clinic. Suffice it to say, the simple appearing process step of "contact the specialist" was extremely complex and time consuming. It was also emotionally exhausting, because each file represented an individual needing care and waiting anxiously for word about their future.

Once a willing specialist was found, making an appointment was relatively easy. However, this often raised timing concerns. The appointment offered might be several weeks, or even months, in the future. Whether the patient could wait that long was another medical decision to be made by a doctor. This required a file review by the Free Clinic Medical Director. This step would appear as a "feedback loop" in a process flowchart, but it was just another complicating factor in the clinic's handling of referrals.

After making an appointment, notifying and getting the patient to the appointment became the next concern. While most Free Clinic patients were grateful, responsible adults, a few were unreliable. Some might not show up for a specialist appointment. Nothing damages the clinic's credibility more than twisting the arm of an over committed specialist and then have the patient be a no show. It is difficult to judge the financial, transportation, and emotional constraints that might have been in play in these cases, but the harm was obvious and it was a process concern. Short of physically delivering the patient to the appointment, the administrative staff had to do everything possible to ensure the patient made the appointment.

Finally, when no specialist could be found, someone had to call the patient and, in effect, tell them, "you're sick, but you're on your own." That is a phone call no one wants to make. It is also a reality of the current health care system because in some cases there is no relief. There is very little that can be done to make this step easier for the clinic or the patient.

The Free Clinic did have an internal referral process in addition to the outside one outlined above. To date, the clinic has offered in-house specialty appointments in three areas – OB/GYN, Orthopedics, and Neurology. Doctors who practiced these specialties had volunteered to serve at the clinic. Some had intended to serve as primary care doctors, taking advantage of the opportunity to practice "front-line medicine" for a change of pace. The medical staff immediately realized that these specialists were resources that must be husbanded and a process for internal referrals quickly developed. It was simple and worked well. The sessions these specialists would be available were identified and appointments restricted to patients needing that care. In other words, a patient could not see a Free Clinic in-house specialist unless first referred during a Free Clinic primary care appointment.

The demand for OB/GYN care was greatest. Patients were listed in a separate log by priority for the next scheduled OB/GYN session. Shortly before the session, an office volunteer would contact the most urgent cases and inform them of their appointment date and time. This revolving patient list might delay an individual's appointment for several weeks, but it was real life triage that ensured the highest-priority cases were seen first. A similar referral procedure applied to Orthopedics, and Neurology, except for the priority step. The lower demand here allowed appointments by a first come, first served basis to work well.

The referral process is another example of how some processes developed and improved as the clinic realized a specific need. Repeating the familiar theme that the clinic planners did not know what they did not know until they began operations, referrals are a perfect example of how processes developed and matured in the first weeks. The referral process was subject to constant improvement, but an optimal state never achieved. The clinic struggled to match demand with resources and could never resolve it. The clinic never gave up on improving the process, but local events brought relief in the form of the Knoxville Academy of Medicine's Knoxville Area Project Access (KAPA). This program alleviated many of the referral worries that the clinic experienced.

The referral process provides an interesting example of unintended consequences. The OB/GYN appointments were outside the regular appointment process. Most office volunteers understood and practiced the correct procedure. However, there is always the small percentage that just doesn't get the word. During some unknown time period, one or more well meaning office volunteers took it upon themselves to schedule OB/GYN appointments whenever a patient called and requested one. (The appropriate response was to ask the patient to come in for a regular appointment and request a referral.)

As a result, some fifteen or so OB/GYN appointments were booked in a session scheduled for six. Twelve patients showed expecting treatment and were accommodated. This meant the doctor and nurse spent twice the time planned at the clinic leaving well after dark. The clinic had to store lab specimens and arrange for a special pickup. In this instance, a volunteer doctor and nurse and a major in-kind donor were needlessly inconvenienced. The clinic had egg on its face that night and the repercussions were severe.

This vignette serves as an introduction to the absolute necessity of quickly developing and promulgating a volunteer handbook. The training that must accompany a handbook is as important as the handbook itself. The JRC insistence on training volunteers before opening day was recalled many times by the steering group during the startup weeks of the Free Clinic. Just as the OB/GYN fiasco hurt the clinic, office staff "free lancing" in other areas had similar results. At times there was little or no consistency in how volunteers interpreted eligibility requirements or applied them. Office volunteers ranged from "strict constructionists" to "laissez faire." There were some unpleasant incidents when office volunteers misapplied the eligibility requirements and summarily turned away patients for minor discrepancies in documentation.

It is probably not fair to blame the office volunteers because they had received very little concrete instruction in the early days. Once the need was comprehended, the planning group worked long and hard to write a volunteer handbook and get it published. The clinic published enough handbooks to give each volunteer a copy and provide one to all new volunteers. Training was made available, but many volunteers had several weeks' service under their belts before publication of the handbook and saw little need for the training. Training should come first and be a requirement for working at the clinic.

This section has attempted to describe in detail several of the areas where trial and error proved to be a reasonable way to develop clinic processes. The clinic staff and the informal steering group realized that constant process improvement would always be necessary. They did not ever believe they had arrived at a final solution to any concern. They only knew the Free Clinic must be a learning organization and seek continual improvement. A final comment on the trial and error process is that it is a necessary step for any clinic. Clinic planners who think they can design a perfect process in advance are mistaken. The fact that improvement will be required should not discourage doing in advance as much as possible, but a realistic expectation that major short falls will be identified during "live" operations must be accepted.

Military planners often say that operation plans are fine until the first shot is fired and then they are of limited practical value. Training and experience must take over. Patient number one is the first shot fired for a new clinic. Anticipate, prepare, plan, but don't be surprised when the clinic staff must go back to the drawing board for a new approach. There is a real tension between over planning and just getting things done. Each start up clinic must find the balance that suits them. They must also accept that constant adjustment, adaptation, improvement, and learning will be part of the journey. This will become most evident when a sufficient amount of experience with actual patients is gained.

THE YEARS

With the first days and weeks behind them, the clinic planners settled into a routine as the clinic became more efficient at handling patients. Most processes were standardized and streamlined where possible. The Foundation continued to provide all financial services for the clinic. The Foundation received all donations and earmarked them for the clinic. The Foundation made most clinic purchases. This relieved the clinic staff of a huge administrative burden. The informal steering committee continued to provide the bulk of the other "office manager" functions. Scheduling doctors, nurses, and office volunteers was a full-time job that often required several phone calls to fill a single requirement. Managing the office volunteers required many on-site hours each week. Reducing all the new and updated procedures to a written, user friendly form for volunteers was a constant activity.

All of these things were accomplished without any full-time staff. Volunteers willing to assume additional responsibilities kept the clinic functioning at a high level. By November 2005, with the clinic open just over three months, the first of many community events took place. November 9th was chosen as the date for what essentially would be a progress report to supporters. The Foundation staff planned a dinner in a Baptist Health System facility located in the clinic neighborhood to update community leaders. It was clear that continuing financial support would be required and The Foundation knew the benefit of quickly publicizing the clinic's positive impact. They hoped that the clinic would be able to report passing the one thousandth appointment milestone. On the night of the event, the Free Clinic had completed approximately 950 appointments and this near achievement of the goal reported.

A PowerPoint slideshow was presented to outline how the clinic was progressing. The period covered was fourteen weeks from August 1 to November 4, 2005. A total of 686 new patients had been treated. Two hundred eight had completed follow-up visits for a total of 894 appointments, or medical encounters. The patients came from fifteen Tennessee counties with the vast majority (75%) from Knox County, the home of the Free Clinic. The percentage of former TennCare patients, based on self-reporting, was forty-one percent. (This figure was of great importance since TennCare, Tennessee's Medicaid program, had recently dropped almost 200,000 individuals from coverage.) Sixty-two percent of patients were female and median age was forty years.

Thirty-three percent of patients had hypertension and twenty-two percent had diabetes (some with both). Prescriptions had been written for 523 patients, many with orders for multiple medications. The clinic had some sample medications on hand and had distributed them to 273 patients. Two hundred seventy-three diagnostic tests had been ordered. The tests were authorized by Baptist Health System, performed by Baptist Hospital, and facilitated and monitored by The Foundation. Eighty-five referrals had been made to specialists. In addition to the sterile numbers, the presentation profiled several specific cases to put a human face on what the clinic was doing.

The clinic had begun not really knowing what to expect in terms of patient load and demographics. How predictive were the first fourteen weeks for the clinic? Some measures have remained steady, most notably county of residence. After forty-three months of operation, the cumulative percentage of patients from Knox County is still seventy-five as it was in November 2005. The number of separate Tennessee counties sending patients is now well over twenty, with one patient from Kentucky. For the life of the clinic, former TennCare patients make up about thirty-eight percent of the patient population. Females continue to out number males with the breakdown settling around fifty-seven percent female. Median age is up to forty-one years, but that includes some patients who were first seen in 2005 and have aged over the years. (Median and average age are calculated using the patient's current age, not the age at first appointment.) Over half of the clinic's patients are hypertensive, diabetic, or both.

In a general sense, the data from the first few weeks were close to describing clinic patients. If there is such a thing as a "typical patient" it was, and has continued to be, a middle aged female from Knox County suffering from high blood pressure or diabetes who has had no health insurance of any sort for most of her adult life.

The number of patients seen, or patient load, was less predictive. For the first three months, the average monthly patient load was 297 medical encounters. For the life of the Free Clinic, the average monthly patient load is 356. In recent months, the monthly patient load has increased dramatically, averaging 416 for the last twelve months. Two of those months had total appointments of over 500 (515 and 511). In short, the Free Clinic has increased its average patient load by forty percent and has every reason to believe it will continue to increase.

In addition to the clinic's report, three additional agenda items merit mentioning. First, the Knox County Mayor was present and presented Dr. Kim with a proclamation declaring a day in recognition of Free Clinic volunteers. The "Knoxville Free Medical Clinic of America Volunteer Day" proclamation acknowledged the service of the over 100 volunteers working at the clinic. The Mayor expressed gratitude for Dr. Kim's long standing community service by providing free medical care, but also identified the new Free Clinic as an important new source of care for the medically underserved. This was a significant step for the Free Clinic because it brought attention to its mission, needs, and accomplishments. Whether directly connected to this event and its report or not, from that time forward the clinic has received some financial support from the Knox County Government.

Second, a Knox County Health Department representative announced plans for a "Dispensary of Hope" pharmacy operation. A Dispensary of Hope collects medicine samples from area doctors and distributes them to needy individuals. This ensures samples don't expire unused and places them in the hands of those who need free medication most. The program had been successful in other cities and planned to open soon in Knox County. Since the Free Clinic was unable to provide medication other than the limited samples it might have on hand, this was welcome news. The dispensary did eventually open and is helping many Free Clinic patients with free medications today. This has helped relieve a major concern of the Free Clinic – how does a cash strapped patient pay for the expensive medication a clinic doctor has prescribed.

Finally, the clinic staff, volunteers, and supporters heard for the first time from Mr. B Ray Thompson, Jr. B Ray is a successful businessman and a passionate philanthropist. He is private and quiet in his giving. He heard of Dr. Kim's work and met him on Father's Day, June 19, 2005. Both Tom Kim and B Ray Thompson have a servant's heart and they talked for four hours at their first meeting. They became fast friends. B Ray is a faithful supporter and his help has been instrumental to the success of the Free Clinic.

This first community report was a success in terms of reporting accomplishments to supporters and providing the staff a better understanding of what the clinic would face over the next few years. In the years that followed, constant improvement was the goal of the clinic staff and it's Board of Directors. The story is rich in detail and could fill many pages. However, only the highlights of the almost four years of clinic operation are covered here. To clarify the narrative, the clinic operational year, August to July, is used rather than a calendar year.

Year One (August, 2005 to July, 2006)

A major milestone was the formation of a clinic board. By November 2005, the clinic had a Board of Directors in place. The board was a good mix of distinguished individuals. It included business people, health care professionals, an attorney, a banker, a CPA, and a local TV news anchor. Wayne Kline, who had done so much to get the clinic started, became chair. The original board had seven members. Over the years it has expanded to twelve. Each new member has brought needed additional skills and expertise.

The board's local standing facilitated the development of broader community support. The dean of local TV news anchors, Bill Williams, was a member of the board. Though retired, he was still an important part of the local media. Through his efforts and other board members, the Free Clinic became relatively well known in the Knoxville area. The clinic usually had both TV and print coverage of any scheduled event such as the November 2005 report to the community. In addition to covering announced events, Dr. Kim and the clinic staff often found themselves interviewed on local or national health care issues. For example, the Michael Moore documentary "Sicko" provided the opportunity for comment. This attention was helpful to the clinic in explaining its mission and letting folks know how they could help.

Because Dr. Kim and other clinic spokespersons are careful not to advocate any particular solution, policy agenda, or political party, the clinic has been successful in keeping the focus on the task at hand. The needs of the uninsured are great and there are many different ways to bring relief. What is important is for each local community to do something. Don't debate policy, just do something! This is an important theme for the Free Clinic. The causes and solution of the current uninsured health care crisis are secondary to helping those in need today. No one will be happier than the Free Clinic volunteers when they are no longer needed. Until that day, they will continue to attack the lack of adequate health care for the uninsured, one patient at a time.

Year one is always difficult for any new non-profit. Regular donors and supporters are not in place and the competition for scarce resources is a fact of life. In the first year of the Free Clinic, The Foundation provided the boost that clearly helped the clinic make it past this first hurdle. The Free Clinic was designated a major recipient of the annual Baptist Health System fund raising event. The "Baptist Nautical Mile" is a well known and well-supported fund raising event in East Tennessee. Announcing major beneficiaries in advance means donors will know who receives their support. To be designated a major recipient not only guarantees a minimum level of financial support, but is an endorsement and validation of the group and its mission. Through the generosity and kindness of The Foundation, the Free Clinic enjoyed both of these benefits during its first year of operation.

Statistically, year one ended with 1,789 individual patients treated. Follow-up visits, returning patients with two or more appointments completed, were 1,109. Appointments, or medical encounters, for the year totaled 2, 898. As a point of clarification, follow-up visits do not necessarily equal the number of patients with multiple visits. Since some patients have many follow-up visits, some as high as fifty, the clinic tracks the number of patients with multiple visits separately. This number is of interest because some grantors want to know how many individuals have made the clinic their medical home – completed two or more visits. For the life of the clinic, approximately forty-five percent of patients have two or more visits.

The value of the "medical home" measure is open to debate. The Free clinic has treated many essentially healthy young working adults who have an episodic complaint such as a cold. They cannot return to work, often in food service, until they can prove treatment and clearance by a doctor. The clinic treats them and provides a standard "return to work" note. Many will not return with another complaint for many years. The clinic has performed a valuable community service, but cannot claim a medical home patient. In this case, the medical home patient measure is not the best indicator of community value as it is in chronic illness cases.

Related is the mix of new to returning patients. On day one, all patients are new. On day two returning patients begin to compete with new patients for appointments. Some area clinics have stopped taking new patients, restricting their service to returning patients. Under this policy, virtually all patients meet the "medical home" criteria. The Free Clinic has never restricted new patients – they compete evenly for appointments with returning patients. The Free Clinic makes appointments as patients call-in without regard to new or old status. The fact that many new patients continue to ask for help seems to be persuasive evidence that the local need for health care for the uninsured remains high.

Year Two (August, 2006 to July, 2007)

The most important event in year two was the closing of Dr. Kim's private practice and his assuming full-time duty as the clinic medical director. He notified his patients well in advance and began the necessary steps to close his practice. There were many "legacy" impacts on the Free Clinic, not the least of which were patients calling the clinic thinking they were talking to "Dr. Kim's office." It took some time, but these issues resolved themselves. Dr. Kim is an extremely compassionate man and he continued to treat some of his elderly patients.

His policy, subject to a few exceptions, was that he would continue to care for individuals over eighty years old and transferred around 100 files to the Free Clinic. In addition to the administrative details, a humorous syntax problem arose when referring to these patients. They were "former" patients of Dr. Kim, but they must also be "old" to qualify. Office volunteers initially asked callers if they were "old" patients which elicited some memorable comments. They then changed to "former" that implied any former Dr. Kim patient was eligible. Either term had its drawbacks, but time and patience resolved the problem.

With Dr. Kim able to spend much more time at the clinic, capacity rose dramatically. During the first year of operation, the monthly average was 240 appointments completed. In the next two years with Dr. Kim full-time, the monthly average was 365 appointments completed. This is a fifty-two percent increase for years two and three over year one. The trend has continued to climb and, after eight months, the monthly average for year four is 450 appointments completed. Since he gave up his private practice, the clinic compensates Dr. Kim as medical director and he became the first paid employee of the clinic. (Technically, he is not an employee, but compensated through a professional personal service contract.)

The Foundation continued to play a key role in the clinic's life throughout year two. Not only did clinic capacity increase with Dr. Kim coming on board full-time, but expenses increased significantly. The Foundation saw the need for financial help and spearheaded the search for funding. It was able to secure grants from both the State of Tennessee and Knox County. As expected, the application process involved significant paperwork, which was completed cheerfully and competently. Both applications were approved and the Free Clinic received, what for it, was significant funding.

In August 2006, the Knoxville Academy of Medicine initiated Knoxville Area Project Access (KAPA). KAPA is a program sponsored by a network of physicians, hospitals, and health care clinics to help those without insurance to obtain the health care services they need. KAPA provides primary care, specialty care, inpatient and outpatient hospital services, mental health services, and prescription drug assistance. KAPA was a Godsend for the Free Clinic because it was overwhelmed by the need for specialty care. The Free Clinic could not find adequate specialty care for its patients.

Dr. Kim and the clinic staff met with the KAPA folks shortly before they began operations and have maintained a cooperative, positive relationship with them ever since. KAPA effectively relieves the burden of finding specialty care for Free Clinic patients. The clinic faxes a referral form to KAPA and in most cases that completes the transaction. KAPA contacts the patient directly and, if qualified, provides the appropriate care. The service could not be better from the Free Clinic's point of view. KAPA assigns a case worker to each patient and follows up on all aspects of treatment.

However, as well as it works, there is a down side to the program. KAPA clients must be residents of Knox County, meaning that twenty-five percent of Free Clinic patients are not eligible for referral. When a patient is not KAPA qualified and a specialist cannot be found through other means, the Free Clinic has the heart-breaking task of informing the patient that there is no free or low cost care available. This is particularly hard because the Free Clinic has usually been the provider of last resort and only an emergency room or other unreasonable solution remains. Even with its limitations, the arrival of KAPA in 2006 marked a turning point for the Free Clinic in that many more patients were successfully referred to specialists.

With the increased patient load, management of workflow, record keeping, volunteer coordination, and running the clinic became more difficult. An obvious solution, deferred for sometime, was to hire a full-time office manager. The clinic planners had wanted to minimize paid staff and rely as much as possible on volunteers, but the tipping point had been reached and hiring a second paid staff member could no longer be delayed. In April 2007, the clinic approached Sandra Brown, a volunteer who had served many hours, and she accepted an offer as full-time office manger. Her Free Clinic experience made the transition almost seamless and in a matter of days all concerned were certain hiring an office manager was the right choice.

The clinic did not realize how important an office manger was until they had one. She assumed duties previously spread among many volunteers. She was available to handle the minor administrative problems that arise and to answer questions of office volunteers. To say that clinic operations became smoother would be an understatement. She was so efficient and willing that she was soon assuming duties far beyond the scope of her job description. She worked closely with Dr. Kim releasing him from many administrative tasks that allowed him to concentrate on treating patients. (The Free Clinic continued to rely heavily on The Foundation and the office manager was technically an employee of The Foundation with her duty station at the clinic.)

As new workflow procedures developed an obvious choke point was identified. Dr. Kim had personally collected and processed all blood test specimens to ensure the highest quality standards. As the number of patients increased, the number of required blood tests increased. Dr. Kim could no longer manage both, so the clinic sought a highly qualified phlebotomist. The Knoxville Academy of Medicine could provide one on an hourly basis and this proved to be a workable solution. The clinic scheduled a phlebotomist for morning hours three days a week and conducted all blood testing at those times. This improved both patient handling and booking appointments.

Dr. Kim closely monitored the drawing of blood and would assist in difficult cases. Still, the contract phlebotomist operation allowed him to concentrate on treating patients. With an office manager to take on administrative duties and relief from the time consuming task of collecting blood samples, Dr. Kim was not only available more hours, but could now devote most of that time to patient care. These three factors (Dr. Kim full-time, hiring an office manager, and a contract phlebotomist), all introduced in year two, made the extraordinary increase in patient load possible.

Statistically, year two ended with 1,693 individual patients treated and 2,455 follow-up visits. Appointments, or medical encounters, for the year totaled 4,148. Cumulative totals were: 3,482 individual patients, 3,564 follow-up appointments, and 7,046 total medical encounters for the life of the clinic.

Year Three (August, 2007 to July, 2008)

The third year of the clinic brought the most significant changes in organization and operations. The first two years had been the clinic's adolescence and young adulthood. The Free Clinic had prospered and grown through the help of many individuals and organizations. These same folks had held the clinic by the hand, taking care of many of the legal, financial, and fundraising tasks faced by most new non-profits. The most apparent of these partners was The Foundation. It had received and disbursed all funds, purchased all supplies, paid all employees, and been involved in virtually every facet of administratively running the clinic.

Local media had reported a possible merger of Baptist Health System for several months in 2007. On January 1, 2008, the merger of Baptist Health System into the newly formed Mercy Health Partners became official. As a result of the merger, The Foundation reorganized into a new entity, Mercy Health Partners Foundation. The impact on the clinic was immediate and far reaching. For clear and fair reasons, this curtailed the support of The Foundation. The Free Clinic would have to grow up and do more things on its own. It was time for the Free Clinic to become a more mature organization.

Neither Mercy Health Partners nor its foundation abandoned the Free Clinic. Their commitment remained high and generous support services such as diagnostic testing at Baptist Hospital (now known as the Riverside Campus) were still provided. However, the reduced staff of the new foundation required a reevaluation of the day to day services it could provide. Among the specific support lost was the grant application and reporting functions and employment services. The clinic must manage future grants as a 501(c) (3) organization. There was sufficient time available to prepare for these eventualities. The clinic opened a bank account to receive and disburse funds and took other steps to face life without the "training wheels" of The Foundation.

Because of the application cycle, The Foundation was able to complete both state and county grant applications for year three before reorganizing. Both were approved. This gave the clinic staff some breathing space for the next cycle. The clinic did not realize how important an office manager was until they had one. That position became more important with the transfer of duties from The Foundation to the clinic staff. Unfortunately, the clinic lost their office manager in June of 2008 when she moved from Knoxville. It was back to square one for the clinic staff as they tried to wrestle with the increased administrative demands and a vacant office manager position. As always, the volunteers rose to the occasion and bridged the gap. The clinic emerged stronger for the experience.

In addition to the challenge of learning to do more with less, the clinic ventured out in two new areas. The first centered on federal funding. The clinic had always tried to avoid anything that smacked of particular health care agendas or politics. However, substantial funding was available to "federally qualified" clinics. The requirements for qualification included a sliding scale fee, so a free clinic could not qualify. If this requirement could be lifted, many additional clinics might be eligible for federal funds including the Free Clinic.

With some local assistance, Dr. Kim was able to obtain a meeting in Washington DC with the appropriate agency. During a one day trip, he met for several hours with the individuals directly responsible for the program and presented the case for including free clinics. He was well received, but unsuccessful. While sympathetic to Dr. Kim's reasoning, they felt the program's intent was clear and the criteria reasonable. They saw no possibility of a change.

The second focused on public awareness of the uninsured. The clinic launched a project that it hoped would have national impact. In October of 2007, a rally was held at the Knox County Department of Health with the dual purpose of bringing attention to the plight of the uninsured and testing support for a bus trip to Washington DC. The purpose of the DC trip would be to simply draw attention to the estimated 50 million uninsured Americans. Awareness is the first step in solving any problem and that was the intention of the riders. It was a call to wake up to reality on a national level. Once convinced of the need, local communities could fashion their own solutions best suited to their situation.

The Free Clinic felt it had two important contributions to make to a national awareness effort. First, it had a workable operational model. The Free Clinic had sprung almost spontaneously from the perceived need in Knoxville and had thrived. It had learned as it grew and was willing to share that experience with others. Second, the clinic could put a human face on the cold hard statistics that make up a large part of the argument for uninsured health care services. Fifty million Americans without health insurance is a concept that is hard to grasp and internalize. Fifty Free Clinic patients willing to ride a bus for twenty hours and tell their story is a more personal and perhaps more powerful concept. Many Free Clinic patients were ready, willing, and able to make the commitment to ride.

The story of the DC trip is rather unique and its full impact as yet unknown. The April 2008 trip included a gathering on the Capitol steps with a banner reminding Americans of the 50 million citizens without health insurance. A local television reporter accompanied the riders, blogging and filming during the twenty-four hours on the bus and in DC. Local TV and print media coverage was very positive and the event met planners' objectives. The riders enjoyed the experience and for some it was their first visit to Washington. The camaraderie of the riders can be measured by the fact that a Dutch treat anniversary dinner in 2009 drew three-quarters of the veterans.

The trip inspired the core group of riders to form a new non-profit, "Clinics of Hope USA" with the mission of planting clinics similar to the Free Clinic. Clinics of Hope could be described in some ways as a spin-off of the Free Clinic, but is an entirely separate entity with a separate mission. The clinics it starts will not necessarily be carbon copies of the Free Clinic, but will have the same goal of providing health care to the uninsured. How that goal is achieved must, and will, vary in different communities. It appears the first "new" clinic may open as soon as the Fall of 2009.

Statistically, year three ended with 1,389 individual patients treated and 3,235 follow-up visits. Appointments, or medical encounters, for the year totaled 4,614. Cumulative totals were: 4,871 individual patients, 6,789 follow-up appointments, and 11,660 total medical encounters for the life of the clinic.

Year Four (August, 2008 to July, 2009)

The learning and adjustments of year three prepared the clinic to move into its fourth year of operation with some confidence. On its own, the clinic was able to apply for and receive both state and county grants. These grants were for Fiscal Year 2009, ending in June 2009, and reflected the downturn in the economy the entire nation was experiencing. The clinic initially was allocated just slightly more than one-half the funds received in FY 2008. This was a serious financial blow and required some adjustments. Late in the fiscal year, the state provided additional funding, probably received as part of the federal stimulus package, and allowed the clinic to close the operational year in better financial shape than expected.

However, patient service was still the driving force and prudent decisions to enhance patient services were not avoided. Foremost among these was the decision to hire a new office manager. The clinic had learned that it could not function effectively without an office manager. This was clearly a "program service" expense and not "overhead," regardless of how an accountant might classify it. A new office manger, Peggy Coley, reported for work in August of 2008 and has proved to be an asset in every way.

A clinical nurse position had been high on the list of clinic needs since opening. The need was obvious and the greater concern was finding an individual suited to the position requirements. Once again, a volunteer with some experience at the clinic expressed an interest. His professional qualifications were impressive, to include experience as a phlebotomist. His needs and the needs of the clinic matched perfectly and a part-time position was created. The clinic could offer regular blood testing three days a week and have an experienced RN on duty.

Both positions required that the clinic assume the duties and responsibilities of an employer. Because The Foundation had handled employment in the past, these were new requirements, but quickly mastered. The clinic staff is also learning more about fund raising, since it can no longer rely on The Foundation to meet this time consuming task. With a paid staff of two full-time and one part-time, the Free Clinic feels well positioned to continue its mission of serving the uninsured in East Tennessee.

A hallmark of the Free Clinic had long been that it served the "Working Uninsured." This was first among its eligibility requirements. The clinic had no apologies for this requirement because experience had shown that demand in this population far exceeded supply. The Free Clinic had early decided to serve this niche and had a full plate with just the employed. However, as the economic downturn worsened, the clinic decided to include the "recently laid-off" as eligible. This allowed established patients to continue treatment at the clinic and softened the blow for many who had lost both a job and health insurance. This policy remains in effect and is indicative of the clinic's desire to be relevant to its community in changing times. This policy has increased the clinic workload and is being absorbed by willing workers.

As of July mid month, the projected yearend statistics for year four are 1,882 individual patients treated and 3,936 follow-up visits. Appointments, or medical encounters, for the year will total 5,818. Cumulative totals expected: 6,753 individual patients, 10,725 follow-up appointments, and 17,478 total medical encounters for the life of the clinic.

THE LESSONS

After forty-four months of operation, the Free Clinic has learned, and continues to learn, many lessons. The knowledge and experience gained during its journey may be helpful to other groups considering community service through a medical clinic. The Free Clinic's history is not necessarily a model to follow, but rather presented as one venture that may have value for others with a similar goal. There are many positive elements that might work well in other situations. There also are many bumps along the road, some of which may be avoided when understood.

The primary lesson is the theme of this story – committed individuals can accomplish a great deal when they decide to just get the job done. Don't do it on the cheap, don't do it on the fly, and don't do it on the margins. Do it right, <u>but do it</u>. There will always be many reasons not to try what will seem an impossible task. Take some risks and get out of the comfort zone. Only through persistence and dedication will

America find an interim solution to the health care crisis. Make no mistake, short term solutions are required. There is no doubt that five, ten, or more years from now health care will be delivered in a radically different manner in America.

But, how will the current uninsured find adequate health care in the time it will take to fully implement some new system? Today's need is overwhelming and action is required now. Unless individuals and organizations are willing to do what they can now, millions of Americans will continue to suffer with less than satisfactory health care. Let those tasked with the responsibility debate the merits of the various health care proposals. That is their job and they are serious, well-intended folks. Others must be willing to tackle another important task at hand – providing immediate relief to those slipping through the cracks.

Another vignette illustrates the point. During a meeting with a high ranking government official, Dr. Kim tried to define the existing need and possible solutions. The official, rather patronizingly, said he did not know much about health care delivery, but that he had staff members who did. Dr. Kim, who was in a wheelchair awaiting back surgery and not his normal congenial self, responded abruptly, "Yes you do. Just start a free clinic in your hometown."

Dr. Kim and the clinic staff were not asking for government assistance. They were not promoting a particular policy or plan. They had no political agenda or party allegiance. They just wanted everyone to realize the breath and depth of the needs of the uninsured in America and be willing to do what they could. Everyone, including this elected official, could do something. An individual of his stature could easily champion a local group to start a single clinic in an area where there was obviously a current need. (Dr. Kim was treating numerous patients from the area that made a long trip to the Free Clinic.) Dr. Kim did not expect the impossible, but he wanted individuals to understand the need and take some appropriate action. He wanted others to be willing to do what they can, and not leave a solution to others or ignore the problem.

Dr. Kim challenged the official to be a clinic champion because that was another important lesson learned. Someone has to be the moving force behind an enterprise as demanding as opening a new community health clinic. There must be a rallying point for the effort. Someone must keep the initial group motivated and focused. If a well-known and influential individual assumes this role, the task is much easier. He or she will draw others to the project and will probably have the skills and abilities to effectively organize them. However, in the final analysis, will is probably more important than any other asset. The champion must be willing to persevere against many difficulties and provide the leadership to reach the group's goal. Most clinics' stories tell of multiple champions, not just an individual.

The original champion can be the center around which multiple champions coalesce. This was the Free Clinic's experience. Dr. Kim is clearly the founding or first champion of the clinic. He had the vision and sought others to help. Wayne Kline emerged as a champion early on, supervising a myriad of legal, business, and organizational details. The vision could not have become reality without the detailed work he carried out. Laura Lee Needham arrived on the scene later, but functioned as a champion. She was the COO of the clinic from day one and continued to serve that role in the critical first months. She was a champion of the clinic by virtue of her commitment, can do attitude, and selfless contribution of time and energy. To single out these three as champions does not diminish the contributions of others. Many individuals contributed significantly to the clinic. Rather, it points out that any new clinic will need one or more persons to be a champion and those individuals must be willing to meet the heavy demands of that role.

With The Foundation's role in opening the clinic so great, why not recognize it as a champion? It is not an oversight. The Foundation was a partner with the Free Clinic from the very beginning. Trying to distinguish between a "champion" and a "partner" could be a semantic nightmare. For very limited purposes, the difference between the two may be that champions "see" and partners "do." Dr. Kim <u>saw</u> a clinic serving the working uninsured. He needed help to do it. The Foundation, working as a partner, was ready, willing, and able to <u>do</u> what it took to field an operating clinic.

With this imprecise distinction of terms, The Foundation was the first of several partners that were instrumental in the success of the Free Clinic. Its contributions, which were the combined efforts of many talented individuals, have been explained. Without the partnership of The Foundation, the clinic probably would never have opened. The Baptist Health System, Baptist Hospital, and subsequently Mercy Health Partners, were also partners in the clinic. They were unstinting in their material and other contributions to the clinic. The Laboratory Corporation of America was an important partner, doing much through in-kind donation of services. Finally, B Ray Thompson, Jr. must be acknowledged as a clinic partner.

The success of any clinic rests on willing partners. A clinic must seek partners and bring them into a real partnership with the clinic. Partners usually have resources that the clinic needs. The clinic and partner goals must be closely aligned. Partners often will see their own goals accomplished by assisting the clinic.

For example, the Free Clinic has a special small business partner who assists with office machine maintenance and repair. In its first few operating days the clinic needed a replacement cartridge for its printer. Since the $90.00 going rate at office supply stores was a big deal to the new clinic, a staff member went to a local business that recycled cartridges. He bought a replacement and in general conversation told the clinic's story. The next day, the clinic received a call from the store's management offering to supply as many cartridges as needed free of charge and to repair any equipment. They just liked the notion that the clinic helped the working uninsured and as a small business recognized the contribution this made to the community. The partnership has continued to the present.

Partners are just one form of community support. The clinic planners knew that wide based community support would be necessary if the clinic were to succeed. This support was built by reaching out to the community to let them know the clinic was there and what it did. The Foundation had public relations experience and helped by preparing materials that could tell the clinic story effectively. The favorable media coverage that the clinic enjoyed has been described. All of these means publicized the clinic and increased support.

However, the clinic staff soon learned that the most loyal and effective promoters of the clinic were its patients. Even in today's 24/7 media world, word of mouth proved the single best means of communicating and building support. Thousands of patients were satisfied clients and over the years their personal endorsements proved their worth. Most patients told several other individuals about the clinic and this included family, friends, coworkers, employers, church members, and others. Most expressed deep gratitude.

The message spread throughout the community. Many small donors appeared at the clinic explaining that the clinic cared for a friend or family member. Church groups called asking for someone from the clinic to share its story. Elected officials heard from constituents. Reporters from small neighborhood newspapers asked for interviews. All these marked the growth of community support that included much more than the original planners, volunteers, supporters, and patients. For every clinic, the wider the base of support is the better.

One key to gaining this support is to concentrate on the mission of helping the sick and, whenever possible, to avoid the rancor often associated with health care policy proposals and the related politics. Every public endeavor has its pitfalls. Health care is particularly prone. Some say Social Security is the "third rail" of political discourse. (Touch this issue and it can potentially kill you.) There are third rails in health care. Universal coverage, socialized medicine, public option, and a host of other terms will spark a debate almost anywhere. Often the debate will have more heat than light. Avoid these arguments by explaining the clinic just helps those who are in need now.

The clinic quickly learned the absolute necessity of volunteer support. Most non-profits must have volunteer support to survive. Since health care by definition is labor intensive, a medical clinic seems to demand more volunteers per client than most. In some sessions, six clinic staff served twelve patients or one staff person per two clients. The average ratio at the clinic is now closer to one staff person per four patients. These ratios point out the necessity for a large volunteer base. Any clinic should test and verify the availability and commitment of its volunteer base early in the planning phase.

Not surprisingly, doctors are the critical component of the volunteer base. Doctors deliver the medical care offered by the clinic. All other volunteers support their efforts. Securing sufficient doctors to cover the hours the clinic is open for patient appointments is the first order of business. Doctors are normally the best recruiters of other doctors for volunteer service. The larger the pool of doctors willing to work at a clinic the better. Alternatives, such as certified physician assistants and nurse practitioners, should be considered. However, these positions may require MD supervision and are usually limited in the services and procedures they may perform.

Doctors are not only the best recruiters for other doctors, but in the Free Clinic's experience proved to be excellent recruiters of nurses. Many doctors volunteering at the clinic chose to bring a nurse from their private practice to serve with them. Most doctors have numerous contacts with nurses and if they are enthusiastic about the clinic can be great spokespersons for the clinic with potential volunteers. Of course, nurses are also great at introducing the clinic to their associates. The Free Clinic also benefited from a retired physician who assumed responsibility for scheduling volunteer doctors. Likewise, a nurse coordinated and recruited nurses whenever possible.

Office volunteers were the third leg of the volunteer triad. In terms of numbers and hours to cover, office workers were the largest volunteer requirement. At least two were needed during patient treatment sessions. At least one was on duty whenever the clinic was open for taking appointments. Again, the clinic staff learned, the larger the pool, the better. It was also clear that "regulars" preferred working a routine schedule. The "Monday morning" and the

"Tuesday afternoon" team of office volunteers that quickly emerged are examples of this notion. These teams simplified scheduling, but did have some drawbacks. When a team or team member was not available to cover their normal day and time, it was often hard to find replacements. Anticipate the need for backups and fill-ins. Again, a large pool makes meeting all your volunteer commitments more likely.

At the same time, the Free Clinic learned that paid staff can be a "force multiplier." When the first office manager was hired, immediate improvement in volunteer performance as noticed. On the job training became more practical and the no-notice cancellation of a nurse or office volunteer was not the problem it would have been before. Volunteers now had someone to answer questions, were happier, and more productive. The consistency in operations improved with on-site supervision of diagnostic testing and referral transactions. The same relief and improvement accompanied the arrival of the current Office Manager.

The same applies to the new RN/Phlebotomist position. This is still a part-time position but it contributes greatly to the efficiency and effectiveness of the clinic. By careful scheduling and management of blood testing, the clinic sees more patients, both for testing and regular appointments. The Free Clinic's success with paid office manager and RN positions is clear and the clinic would probably have been better served by filling them earlier. Personnel costs are high, but select positions can be worth far more than their cost.

Five Fingers

A lesson brought home several times was that a new volunteer clinic must never appear to be in competition with any other health care provider, private or public. It should serve a niche or unmet need. A new clinic probably cannot meet its own particular client demands, whether they are working uninsured, homeless, or any other category. The health care need is so great that, for the present, there will always be room for a new clinic. Also, many look to government to fill the health care needs of its citizens, citing some form of public health care as a standard for an industrialized nation. Someday this may be a reality. In the interim, which some people think will be years if not decades, there is a need for volunteer clinics of every sort. Most volunteer clinics look forward to the day when they can say, "We worked ourselves out of a job," but in the meantime there is plenty of work for all.

Every new clinic will face some opposition. The Volunteers in Medicine (VIM) Clinic on Hilton Head Island, South Carolina is an example. Dr. Jack B. McConnell, the founder, was featured on the *Today* show in July 2007 and is an icon in the volunteer health care community. As detailed in his book <u>Circle of Caring: The Story of the Volunteers in Medicine Clinic</u>, it took two and a half years of hard work before the clinic opened on July 5, 1994.

The need for health care for the uninsured is great, but that does not mean every local solution will be the same. There is no "one size fits all" approach to a community health clinic that will work everywhere. The Knoxville Free Clinic had some special support that made it possible to develop its very lean operation. Baptist Hospital was close by and could provide support that might not be available to a new clinic in another location or situation. The fact that the clinic operated almost in the shadow of a partner hospital made its specific methods possible. A clinic located in a rural area might, and probably will, have to consider including X-rays, basic lab work, and a pharmacy of some sort on site.

The lesson is simply that cookie cutter clinics are not always feasible. The Free Clinic learned that it could not be a clone of other area, regional, or national clinics. Each clinic must adapt to its environment and the special conditions that surround it. In many ways, any new clinic must find its special niche. Niche is an overused marketing word, but it captures what clinic planners should do. They must find the "space or gap" in the local uninsured health care "market" that is not being filled by other providers and set out to fill it. Then they will not compete with existing providers, but complement them by identifying and meeting an unmet need.

When possible, dental needs should be addressed by clinic planners. A sad fact is that, when evaluating unmet needs, dental care will often be at the top of the list. One accepted estimate is that, while fifty million Americans lack health insurance, a staggering 100 million receive no basic dental care. The Free Clinic learned that, at least in numbers of patients seeking care, dental may be the greater need. Working cooperatively on two Remote Area Medical

(RAM) interventions reinforced this notion for the Free Clinic staff.

RAM, founded by Stan Brock of TV's *Wild Kingdom* fame, organizes medical activities internationally and throughout the United States, concentrating on underserved areas. Medical, dental, and optometry services are typically provided on a first come first served basis. Requests for dental service normally outweigh all others.

The Free Clinic has numerous current and potential clients who are searching for dental care. Initially, the clinic could not meet this need and all these patients were referred to other local dental providers. These providers might not qualify them for dental care; and, when they do, there may be very long waiting periods. To bring some relief, Dr. Kim researched the option of performing simple extractions at the Free Clinic.

He found the clinic could perform extractions and, with training and equipment provided by RAM, he began to make simple extractions. Again, caution was the overriding principle. He took on only the simplest cases, described in his words as "the tooth must be ready to fall out." He was obviously well qualified to prescribe and administer antibiotics, which usually were clearly indicated and brought immediate relief. Dental care is an important concern and when possible should be included in clinic services.

Recognizing the need for change was another reality the clinic staff had to understand. The original plans for the clinic could not foresee all the eventualities of the next four years. Things change and the clinic had to be ready to adapt. The clinic opened with fairly regular evening and Saturday sessions. These went well for about a year and were appreciated by patients. However, after the first year, the doctors providing the primary coverage of these blocks were no longer available. The clinic calendar had to adjust and those sessions curtailed. The clinic still has occasional evening sessions, but not with the regularity of the first year. The clinic does not currently schedule Saturday sessions.

Another major change was the loss of free radiologist services. The standard practice for imaging diagnostics such as X-rays, etc., is to bill separately for the imaging and reading by a radiologist. Initially, Free Clinic patients received both totally free and involved no bill for either service. After some time, the donor radiology practice decided it could no longer continue to provide the free service. Knowing how generous the radiology practice had been already made negotiating hard for the clinic staff. How do you ask those who have already given so much for more? However, the clinic did ask for relief and the doctors agreed to perform the service for clinic patients at thirty percent of the standard fee. This dramatically changed operating procedures for diagnostic testing, but patients and staff seemed to adapt well. Again, any clinic must be ready to adapt to changing requirements and the additional burdens they may impose.

When major chain pharmacies introduced "$4 generic" prescriptions, the clinic cheerfully adjusted.

By placing a copy of the standard formulary from each store in the exam rooms, clinic doctors were able to write many prescriptions that patients could have filled for $4, which was normally within their ability to pay. This one change brought a great deal of relief to clinic patients. In the past, many patients would have a prescription, but no way to pay for it. Clinic staff often pulled cash from their own pocket to encourage patients to get the medicines they needed. With $4 generics, those days are almost gone.

The clinic had always required patients, or spouses/parents, be employed. As explained, the clinic felt this was a fair and rational requirement and uniformly enforced throughout the life of the clinic. As the economic downturn deepened and more folks lost their jobs, it seemed reasonable to suspend the employment requirement. The clinic amended the requirement to include recently laid off as well as employed. Patients must document this status just as they document employment. This illustrates adjustment to changing conditions, and one perceived by most as in favor of patients.

Among other lessons learned was the obvious one that no clinic can be everything to everybody and that often there is no choice but to say no. The most emotionally challenging of these situations is when patients call, or come in, expecting emergency room attention. The Free Clinic is simply not staffed or equipped to handle any true emergencies. To do anything other than to direct the individual to the nearest ER or to call 911, is taking a huge risk for both the person and the clinic. Volunteers need the training to say no and to be firm, even when a distraught mother is describing a child's pain and begging for help. For office volunteers who are the front line for phone calls and walk-ins, knowing what the clinic can't do is as important as knowing what the clinic can do.

Another lesson is to beware of strings. Some individuals and organizations will offer gifts that have strings attached. Many grants will have operational and funding requirements that are onerous to your clinic. The point is to keep your eyes open and read the fine print of any offer. Many grantors expect that they are giving funds to a large, well-equipped operation, not a small paper operation like the Free Clinic. Clinic planners or staff should address these concerns directly with any potential donor. In one case, support offered the Free Clinic required reporting using standard medical practice software that the clinic did not have. The Free Clinic staff explained why they could not comply. Much to their surprise and delight, the requirement was waived and the support delivered.

A final lesson may be "If you build it, they will come." This line from the movie *Field of Dreams* is an expression of the great need in this country for some way to care for the uninsured. There is no doubt that at the present time there are millions of unserved and underserved working uninsured. It seems it would be hard to find a place where, if a clinic opens, the uninsured would not line up at the door on day one. It is probably possible that there are such places and that is why a needs survey is required. A needs survey gives the best chance of putting a clinic that offers

Five Fingers

the right services in the right place and will give the highest ROI.

Realizing that the need is so great and our country so far behind in providing care should encourage some walking by faith. The working uninsured are generally very proud people and rarely complain or directly ask for help. It is not clear that their needs are always fully captured in the statistical nets cast by social researchers. No one wants to wait a year for the extraction of an abscessed tooth. No one wants to wait a month to get a refill of their hypertension medication. So, when a new clinic for the uninsured opens, it is a good bet they will come.

NOW WHAT?

The lessons learned and being learned by the Free Clinic completes this story of a new community clinic in Knoxville, Tennessee. It took about six months from vision to opening. The goal was not to open quickly, but rather not to be deterred and delayed by the obstacles encountered along the way. This mission oriented attitude allowed the clinic to rapidly move through the many milestones necessary to open a clinic. The call to immediate action was more than a mantra; it was a philosophical approach to how to do business. Do it right, but take some risks.

Now that the story has been told, so what? What was the purpose of detailing the many aspects of clinic planning and operation covered so far? The answers to those questions are simple. The objective of the exercise is to encourage others to make the same journey. Not necessarily to follow the same path, but to head out for the same destination. To recap, the needs of the uninsured are huge and will remain so for some time. Until the plight of the uninsured in America is adequately addressed, grassroots efforts to provide local solutions will be required. Every clinic that opens is a step in the right direction, whether it provides a medical home for 50, 500, 5,000, or many more.

Now is the time for action. This was not the time for analysis paralysis. Waiting for a government or other solution is not a viable alternative. Bridging the gap between today's reality and tomorrow's promise is a necessity. Yesterday was the time to open a clinic serving a neglected segment of our population – the millions without adequate medical care. Virtually everyone involved in the volunteer community health clinic movement, wants to work themselves out of a job. They see their mission as a temporary one; again, bridging a gap. How long that gap will persist is unknown, and that is why it is important to bring more clinics on-line quickly.

The KISS (Keep It Simple, Stupid) principle may be one way to bring more capacity online quicker. Health care for the uninsured can be kept simple, without sacrificing quality. As noted, a physician seeing just one patient in the office for free is a start. This ensures a high level of care in an existing setting that requires little or no additional material support. The doctor gives the care for free and a nurse may volunteer to assist. No BIR support is required because there is no billing or insurance. As in the first iteration of the Free Clinic, this is a no muss, no fuss operation.

Dr. Kim's Briceville free clinic, which is still in operation, is another example. This clinic is little more than Dr. Kim showing up with his stethoscope. This is not to trivialize what he does or to imply that less than high practice standards are met. However, when the treatment is limited, the support required can be limited. If the Free Clinic is analogous to a battalion aid station, the Briceville clinic would be a company medic. Just as casualties are evacuated through the military medical system until they reach a facility capable of the level of care they need, the same takes place in this example. Dr. Kim has referred Briceville patients to his own Knoxville Free Clinic when the situation warrants because he has more support there. Some of those patients moved on to specialists, including at least one case of major surgery which Kim was able to arrange. A willing doctor with a stethoscope and prescription pad operating out of a loaned storefront can be the beginning of a new clinic.

Opening a clinic is not rocket science. It is hard, demanding, meticulous work, but not beyond the ability of dedicated, motivated groups. The will to do it is the most important requirement. Appendix I provides some sources of additional information for interested individuals. Those who choose to start their own journey will find it is worth every bit of the time and other resources required. And, it has its own special rewards, for as has been said, "In healing others, we heal ourselves."

Appendix I - Additional Information

For additional information about the need for clinics to assist the uninsured or for assistance starting, operating, or expanding a community clinic, please contact:

The Free Medical Clinic - A Christian Ministry
6209 Chapman Highway
Knoxville, Tennessee 37920
Phone: (865) 577-3733
E-mail: freemedicalclini@bellsouth.net
Website: www.freemedicalclinic.net

Volunteers in Medicine Institute
162 St. Paul Street
Burlington, Vermont 05401
Phone: (802) 651-0112
E-mail: info@vimi.org
Website: www.volunteersinmedicine.org

Clinics of Hope, USA
E-mail: healthcareaccessgroup@yahoo.com
Website: www.healthcareaccessgroup.org

Remote Area Medical Foundation
1834 Beech Street
Knoxville, Tennessee 37920
Phone: (865) 579-1530
E-mail: ram@ramusa.org
Website: www.ramusa.org

National Association of Free Clinics
P. O. Box 151352
Alexandria, Virginia 22315
Phone: (571) 243-3632
E-mail: info@freeclinics.us
Website: www.freeclinics.us

About the Author

Tom Kim

Dr. Tom Kim was born in North Korea. His family settled in the United States and Tom completed high school and college in Indiana and Tennessee. After graduation in 1969, he returned to Korea for medical school and received his MD in 1974. After four years additional training in the United States, he accepted a fellowship in Hematology and Oncology at the University of Tennessee Medical Center in Knoxville. He has been in private practice in Knoxville since 1981.

Motivated by a deep sense of gratitude to his adopted land and the Lord's command to "Love your Neighbor," Dr. Kim began serving the working uninsured in an after-hours clinic in his medical office. In 2005, Dr. Kim led an effort to greatly expand this service into a full-time facility with over 100 volunteer doctors, nurses, and office workers. Today the clinic, also known as The Free Medical Clinic – A Christian Ministry, serves over 6,500 uninsured patients, a number which continues to grow as new patients discover the clinic.

Dr. Kim also has been recognized locally and nationally for his work honoring and supporting Korean War veterans.

Ed Cate

Ed Cate is a retired Army officer and office volunteer at the Free Clinic.

LaVergne, TN USA
18 November 2009
164555LV00001B/1/P